Sport and Alcohol

There is a clear sense in which sport has played, and continues to play, an important role in the normalization and legitimization of routine, excessive and problem drinking; sport and alcohol have become inextricably linked. Alcohol companies provide funding in the form of sponsorship, fans consume alcohol when watching, and players celebrate, bond and relax with alcohol. *Sport and Alcohol: an ethical perspective* aims to critically examine the various ways in which sport and alcohol interact.

In doing so, the book casts an ethical eye over the following topics:

- society's relationship with alcohol
- sponsorship and marketing of alcohol through sport and its effect on children
- sport's alcohol-tolerant ethos, problematic drinking practices and rituals
- punishment and discipline in relation to athletes' drink-related bad behaviour
- alcoholism in the context of sport and the need for a greater understanding of the condition, how it develops and what can be done
- the status of athletes as role models.

Offering a much-needed critical assessment of an important issue in contemporary sport and society, *Sport and Alcohol* is essential reading for those interested in the social, cultural or philosophical study of sport in general and sport and alcohol in particular.

Carwyn Rh. Jones is Professor in Sports Ethics at the Cardiff School of Sport at Cardiff Metropolitan University, UK. He was formerly president of the International Association for the Philosophy of Sport and a founding member of the British Philosophy of Sport Association. He is co-editor of Routledge's *The Ethics of Sport Coaching* and Cambridge Scholar's *Philosophy of Sport*. He has published widely on a broad range of ethical and sociological issues in sport.

Routledge Research in Sport, Culture and Society

Sport and Alcohol

An ethical perspective

Carwyn Rh. Jones

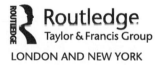

Routledge
Taylor & Francis Group

LONDON AND NEW YORK

First published 2016
by Routledge

2 Park Square, Milton Park, Abingdon, Oxfordshire OX14 4RN
711 Third Avenue, New York, NY 10017

Routledge is an imprint of the Taylor & Francis Group, an informa business

First issued in paperback 2017

British Library Cataloguing-in-Publication Data
A catalogue record for this book is available from the British Library

Library of Congress Cataloging in Publication Data
Names: Jones, Carwyn Rhys.
Title: Sport and alcohol: an ethical perspective/Carwyn R. Jones.
Description: New York: Routledge, 2016. | Includes bibliographical
    references and index.
Identifiers: LCCN 2015036539 | ISBN 9781138807976 (Hardback) |
    ISBN 9781315750804 (eBook)
Subjects: LCSH: Athletes—Alcohol use.
Classification: LCC RC1245 .J66 2016 | DDC 616.86/10088796—dc23
LC record available at http://lccn.loc.gov/2015036539

ISBN: 978-1-138-80797-6 (hbk)
ISBN: 978-1-138-55872-4 (pbk)

Typeset in Times
by Swales & Willis Ltd, Exeter, Devon, UK

I fy mab

Contents

Acknowledgements

Writing this book has been a challenge and there are many people who have contributed directly and indirectly to the process. I am very grateful to Professor Mike McNamee who supervised my doctoral thesis in sport and moral development, and has been a good friend, mentor, advisor, critic and colleague over the last 20 years. I am also grateful to members of the International Association for the Philosophy of Sport and the British Philosophy of Sport Association for providing a warm and stimulating academic environment in which to discuss and develop my ideas. I am indebted to Routledge and in particular to Simon Whitmore and William Bailey for taking on this project. I must also mention Mike McGuinness, Paul Davis, Keir Worth, Lisa Edwards, Scott Fleming, Alun Hardman, Jim Parry, Ian Pritchard, Verner Møller and Hywel Iorwerth, all of whom have played an instrumental role in my career one way or another. Heather Sheridan too, falls into this bracket, but she has also carefully proofread the book and provided invaluable feedback. I also wish to acknowledge Cardiff School of Sport who have afforded me the time and support to undertake this writing task.

On a more personal note, I want to thank Wynford Ellis Owen who helped save my life and my sanity and provided me with love and wisdom, which I can never repay. There are many other friends who share a fellowship that continues to be my anchor. George, one such friend, was courageous enough to allow me to tell his story in this book. I want to thank my parents Alun and Lilian Jones and the rest of my family for their love and forbearance. My deepest gratitude goes to my wife Enlli for her love and support through good and bad times. Finally I want to mention my son Tomos Llywelyn who has brought unimaginable joy and meaning to my life.

Diolch yn fawr – Thank you

Introduction

It speaks volumes for the place alcohol has in our culture that I now get frequent requests to sponsor people to abstain from alcohol for charity. Raising money for charity is of course laudable, but to go without alcohol for a month is surely no great hardship nor particularly noteworthy, especially in comparison to running a marathon or climbing Kilimanjaro.[1] Our culture, however, has an alcohol problem. Many are dependent on alcohol, perhaps not in the sense that they are addicted, but in the sense that alcohol is ever-present. We get anxious if access to it is threatened in some way and feel that abstaining for a month is deemed noteworthy. Alcohol is the compulsory accompaniment to all celebrations, social events, meals and holidays, and it seems we cannot go without it even at events primarily aimed at children. Evidence that alcohol is woven into the very fabric of our society in this way is not difficult to find. In Wales, where I live and grew up, there is a wonderful youth movement called the *Urdd* (The Order). The *Urdd* is a movement, established in 1922, to give children and young people the chance to socialize and learn through the medium of Welsh (the indigenous minority language of Wales). It promotes a number of important values and organizes opportunities to engage in a range of activities including sport and the arts. Every year the *Urdd* organize a peripatetic national festival (Eisteddfod) for children where singing, dancing, recital, arts and crafts and other competitions provide the main focus. Children and their families visit the week-long festival, not only to compete but to socialize among the various stalls, shops and trade stands. Prior to the 2010 festival the *Urdd* decided that, for the first time, they would permit the sale of alcohol on the grounds of the festival field. Of course, the *Urdd* strongly defended their stance, arguing that no alcohol would be sold to anyone under the legal age, but it struck me and others who campaigned against the move that even a festival for children was considered deficient in some important way unless alcohol was available. There are other, perhaps less esoteric, examples. In the UK in 2013 there were over 8000 applications by primary schools for licenses to serve alcohol at fetes, discos and sports days, with some serving 'mocktails' to children, ensuring that they are initiated into the pleasure, ritual and allure of drinking alcohol. According to a report by the Joseph Rowntree Foundation, 40% of 6-year-old children in the UK could identify at least one alcoholic drink by smell alone, rising to 75% by the age of 10.[2]

I believe that alcohol has a grip on society, and, despite the untold negative consequences, it continues to play a central role in our culture. Parents even introduce their children to the substance which is significantly more likely to kill them, and more readily available, than any other drug. Alcohol is not just another commodity. It is a potentially dangerous and toxic substance which produces an altered state. Young people drink to get drunk on nights out and put themselves and others at risk of a range of harms. For fans of alcohol, however, the problems associated with it lie not with the substance itself, but with the character and choices of those who abuse it or cannot handle it. Consequently there is, and always has been, opposition to anti-liberal views or policies which might curtail the freedom of individuals to drink as they choose. Much has been written about alcohol and its sociohistorical role in many cultures and there is a significant literature dealing with a broad range of issues relating to it.

My aim in this book is to focus specifically on some issues that arise in relation to alcohol in the context of sport. I address three broad themes. First, I problematize both sport's role in promoting alcohol through sponsorship and advertising and the drinking ethos which characterizes many aspects of sporting culture. Next, I look at whether we are entitled to criticise athletes as 'bad' role models when it comes to alcohol consumption and related behaviour.[3] Finally, I examine in detail some important questions surrounding punishment, moral responsibility and addiction in relation to athletes who seem to have particular difficulties with alcohol.

Not everyone drinks alcohol and not everyone who drinks alcohol drinks too much, but many do and it causes a number of untold problems. As such, the thrust of my arguments in this book are critical of alcohol and the attitudes and behaviours associated with it. Its supporters and promoters are powerful and there is no shortage of sources selling us the message that alcohol is essential to the good life, not least in the context of sport. In addition to the social benefits of drinking, we are told that it is also good for our health in moderation and might protect us from a host of medical conditions. There seem to be daily, contradictory, misleading and potentially dangerous advice about alcohol's purported benefits. A recent study by Knott et al. (2015) suggests that any health benefits from alcohol may be limited to a small group of people, namely women over the age of 65 years. Even if such benefits were available, it is doubtful that many people drink at the moderate levels suggested and evidence shows that significant percentages drink far too much.

In terms of the perspective this book takes, there are two points to make. The first is about the disciplinary background that informs it. This book applies philosophical method and ethical theory to the issue of sport and alcohol. The second point concerns me as the author. It seems fairly common, particularly in some branches of the social sciences in sport, to say something about the author or to come clean and 'announce bias' so that readers are aware of the author's particular perspective. I am not convinced about the merits of such a practice for reasons expounded by McFee (2010: 94); however, by way of conformity I offer the following information about me which the reader may or may not find interesting or relevant.

I played non-elite rugby from an early age, live in a culture and city where sport and alcohol dominate, know a lot of people who are, or have been involved with, elite-level sport, have read numerous biographies and autobiographies of former elite athletes, work on a UK university campus where alcohol is a routine part of student life and where attendance at lectures on Thursday morning is considered unreasonable given that Wednesday afternoon is match day. I support Liverpool FC and Wales RFU and have for years tacitly endorsed Carlsberg Lager and Brains Bitter by wearing replica kits. I watch sport on television and see the adverts for alcohol and the champagne- and beer-soaked celebrations of athletes. I am also a non-drinker or, perhaps worse still, a reformed drinker. Until the age of 34 I regularly drank alcohol, but realized that I had less and less control over how much I drank once I started. It was a problem which I had to solve. More than nine hangover-free years later I see the world through the eyes of a (growing) minority who do not drink at all (no, not even 'one' at Christmas). I am also a father of a toddler who I hope will not be encouraged, dared, pestered and challenged to drink long before he is old enough to make sensible decisions about alcohol and while his body is susceptible to alcohol's noxious effects. There is perhaps more one might say here, but to paraphrase McFee (2010: 94), there is no way one can offer 'all' the relevant facts about me because there is no finite totality of such facts that any given reader might think relevant.

In terms of structure, Chapter 1 attempts to provide the background to the book. I argue that alcohol is a toxic drug which is taken primarily for its mood-altering property. A consequence, or perhaps a side effect of this characteristic, is that many people misuse or overuse alcohol, which leads to a number of problematic issues. Despite the dangers of alcohol, I argue that it is treated differently to other toxic mood-altering substances and is sold, marketed and promoted by a powerful and influential corporate juggernaut as a life-affirming elixir. Medical experts are largely in agreement that alcohol is a serious problem in contemporary Western society. In many countries, however, the alcohol industry itself is largely responsible for health promotion messages. This is an untenable situation where profit and health are in direct competition.

In the second chapter I argue that sport plays a significant and problematic role in normalizing drinking in general, and excessive or binge drinking in particular, in three ways. First, although there are certain restrictions on alcohol marketing in many countries, sport provides alcohol companies with a vehicle to market and promote their products to current and future consumers. As such, sport plays a key role in introducing children to alcohol brands that are often printed on replica strips, advertising hoardings and racing cars and feature in the names of major tournaments and events. Secondly, I argue that watching 'the game' is an occasion which licenses excessive drinking at home or in the pub and there is clear evidence that such game-related drinking (beyond the risks to the individual) contributes to disorder, aggression and violence (including domestic violence). Finally, I argue that sport encourages or normalizes the alcoholic 'binge'. Excessive drinking is *the* choice for celebration, relaxation or team bonding.

In Chapter 3, I apply the concept of ethos to the issue of sport and alcohol. Drawing on McLaughlin's (2005) idea of ethos as a 'spirit' or 'tone', I develop the idea that many sporting cultures have an alcohol-tolerant ethos at best and an ethos which promotes problematic alcohol use at worst. The picture is mixed and complex, but I push the idea that even where the official line (intended ethos) is hostile to alcohol use (especially at certain times), many players and coaches still see excessive drinking as desirable and acceptable. Despite the 'professional' era and its high expectations in terms of athlete fitness, the evidence shows that some athletes drink at the wrong times, or drink too much on certain occasions. We are bombarded with daily media stories about athletes getting into varying degrees of trouble after drinking. Such an ethos is morally troubling because young athletes are subjected to a culture that normalizes excessive drinking.

In Chapter 4 I examine the line of criticism most often put forward when famous athletes get into trouble through drinking. In such cases they are accused of being bad role models and setting a bad example. I examine more carefully the use of the 'role model' concept in moral evaluations of athletes in general, and of their alcohol-related behaviour in particular. I argue that we are entitled to expect reasonable standards of behaviour from athletes and that we are justified in condemning them when they fail to meet such standards. We are particularly justified in doing so when they get drunk and behave badly because such behaviour has direct and indirect influence on others.

In Chapter 5 I explore the practice of punishing individual players for drink-related behaviour. First, I examine the concept of punishment and its various justifications, focusing specifically on what constitutes offending when it comes to athletes drinking. Second, I examine some of the moral issues associated with punishing someone who is drunk because their autonomy and rational decision-making capacity is severely diminished by alcohol. Finally, I introduce the idea that *the* most important decision in drink-related offending is often the decision to start drinking. Problems arise because many athletes (on certain occasions) set out to get 'plastered'. The widespread and collective intention to drink heavily embedded in the ethos of many sports and beyond must change if the deleterious consequences of intoxication are to be stopped.

In Chapter 6 I focus specifically on a small but very visible minority of athletes who have had serious problems with alcohol addiction. I discuss the concept of addiction and its relationship with free will and autonomy and touch on the implications of addiction as a medical rather than a moral issue. Addiction is a process which can end in the tragic and painful death of an athlete, but starts long before that with behaviour which may or may not be taken as symptomatic of addictive potential. I discuss the difficulties surrounding what should be done about athletes who are exhibiting drink problems.

The final chapter is different from the previous chapters in terms of the methodology and content. It is a life history of a former professional football player who became an alcoholic. My aim in presenting this story is in part a counterpoint to the glamorization of alcoholism associated with superstars like George Best. In the end, George Best died an alcoholic death, yet a prevailing narrative continues to portray a 'playboy star' who liked women and drink and lived life to the full. As we know, the truth about addiction is very different as Best and countless others have revealed in autobiographies which show the ugly, painful and tragic side of the condition. In some cases the families of these addicts have also told their side of the story, which gives a more complete and disturbing picture of the addict (for example, Callum Best's recent biography). This chapter tells the story of 'George' (a pseudonym) and provides an insight into the mindset of an addict before, during and after active alcoholism.

As I mentioned at the start, this is not a sociological text, although it touches on sociological issues. My analysis does not fully address a number of cultural, gender, race and ethnicity issues, but the key arguments do not stand or fall on these concerns. There is also an inevitable UK-centric focus to the book, but the issues covered are by no means exclusively British. While there is a logical sequence to the chapters, the book is not one unfolding argument. There are three or four related arguments which do not necessarily rest on the validity of each other. Although there is evidence that there is a slowing down of the problem of excessive alcohol consumption, with fewer people drinking so much and so often, this book is a timely contribution to the debate.[4] The problems associated with alcohol in sport continue and are considerable.

Notes

1 http://www.theguardian.com/commentisfree/2014/oct/01/sober-october-giving-up-alcohol-not-heroic (accessed 5/05/2015).
2 http://www.theguardian.com/society/2014/mar/08/ban-alcohol-primary-school-events-swanswell?CMP=share_btn_tw (accessed 5/05/2015).
3 I use the referent 'athlete' in this book as a general term for those who play sport of all kinds. It is also a gender-neutral term.
4 http://www.economist.com/news/economic-and-financial-indicators/21636774-alcohol-consumption (accessed 5/05/2015).

References

Knott, C.K., et al., 2015. All cause mortality and the case for age specific alcohol consumption guidelines: pooled analyses of up to 10 population based cohorts. *British Medical Journal*. doi: http://dx.doi.org/10.1136/bmj.h384.

McFee, G., 2010. *Ethics, knowledge and truth in sport research: an epistemology of sport*. London: Routledge.

McLaughlin, T., 2005. The educative importance of ethos. *British Journal of Educational Studies*, 53(3), 306–325.

1 Alcohol and its harms

Introduction

In this chapter, I provide a brief background to the rest of the book. Alcohol is a toxic mind-altering (psychoactive) drug that causes a number of problems. The extent of harms and costs incurred by many societies and individuals as a result of alcohol testifies to its widespread use and abuse. Despite the risks associated with alcohol, its consumption is at the centre of many cultural practices and traditions, including watching and playing sport, and there is significant resistance to policies infringing our freedom to buy and consume it. Our positive, or at least tolerant, attitudes towards alcohol are entrenched and come into sharp relief when we compare alcohol with other psychoactive drugs; alcohol laws in many countries are liberal in comparison to those governing other psychoactive substances. There is strong resistance to a change of policy in light of scientific evidence and alcohol industries play a powerful role in resisting changes that would affect profits.

Alcohol: no ordinary commodity

Alcohol has always played a central role in a variety of different cultural practices. It has been consumed for intoxication purposes (to get drunk), but has also been used for medicinal, symbolic and ritualistic purposes. Despite alcohol's ubiquitous presence in our supermarkets, bars and restaurants, and on our television screens, Babor et al. (2010: 11) argue that alcohol is 'no ordinary commodity'. Although it is bought by consumers regularly, much like other grocery items, it is a drug consumed primarily for its intoxicating rather than nutritional properties. Alcohol, or ethanol (the molecule $CH_3–CH_2–OH$) is similar to other drugs in this respect. Although it might be taken in various forms and flavours, ethanol is ingested 'not for the molecules under that description, but for the molecules because of what they do' (Flanagan 2011: 273). Its universal appeal, its *raison d'être*, lies with (like other drugs) its psychoactive properties; its ability to change the way we feel or bring about an altered state. It does this by directly changing the chemical state of our brains. Alcohol is a drug that has both depressive and stimulating effects. Alcohol stimulates because it activates the gamma-aminobutyric acid (GABA) receptor and depresses because it also releases noradrenaline (norepinephrine).

Consequently, alcohol can relieve anxiety, help with sleep and relaxation, but can also improve sociability, lower inhibitions and lead to a loss of control. There may be many reasons why human beings as a species are so preoccupied with changing mood, but Davenport-Hines (2002: xiv) suggests that 'the use of drugs often reflects other sets of human ideals: human perfectibility, the yearning for a perfect moment, the peace that comes from oblivion'. In a more theistic account, Carl Jung's letter to Bill Wilson, the co-founder of Alcoholics Anonymous (AA), interpreted one of his patients' desire for alcohol, or more precisely the desire for its effect, in the following way: 'His craving for alcohol was the equivalent, on a low level, of the spiritual thirst of our being for wholeness, expressed in medieval language: the union with God' (cited in Flanagan 2013: 80). The corollary of the transformative property of alcohol and other drugs is their power to harm individuals and communities.

The most obvious negative effects of alcohol – getting drunk and losing control – mean that along with its history of production and consumption, it has a history of opposition. According to Nicholls (2009: 2):

> Drink has always existed both as an activity and a set of questions: questions about the rights and wrongs of intoxication, about the role of government in regulating free trade, about the limits of personal freedom, about gender, class, taste and health.

Contemporary concerns about alcohol consumption are nothing new. Different governments or organizations in various countries at different times have, for religious, moral, health, economic and other motives, attempted to paternalistically influence their citizens' alcohol consumption. Legislation, education, moralizing and prohibition have all been used at various times with different levels of success. For example, in the UK, during the Industrial Revolution, alcohol played a significant role in class relations. In terms of crude class control, 'the industrialists exploited the cultural power of alcohol to the fullest extent' by paying the workers in company-owned public houses (Pritchard 2006: 305). Consequently, the men would spend their meagre wages on beer, further exacerbating their reliance on the 'company'. Both the expenditure and the drunkenness would aggravate the already difficult social conditions prevalent at that time. Temperance movements began to emerge to combat the invidious threat of alcohol in order to protect both the souls of the workers and the well-being of their families. Ironically, at the time, drinking beer (fairly weak in comparison to today's standards) had advantages. Water purity was poor and cholera was relatively common. The brewing process purified water and it was often safer to drink beer. More recently, the ever-present threat of drink was described by Asquith, the British Prime Minister before the First World War, as 'a greater threat than Austria and Germany combined' (Nicholls 2009: 1).[1] In the USA, the Volstead Act of 1919 marked the start of a period of prohibition where the manufacture, sale and transportation (but not the consumption) of alcohol became illegal.[2] In addition to the well-known, and arguably infamous, prohibition period in the USA, various forms of restriction and control of alcohol endure. The production and sale of alcohol continues to be regulated to a greater or lesser degree in most countries. A key difference between alcohol and other marketable products, and the reason it is subject to restrictions, is based on the growing evidence which shows 'that alcohol intoxication, alcohol dependence, and the toxic effects of alcohol on various organ systems are key mechanisms linking alcohol consumption to a wide range of adverse consequences' (Babor et al. 2010: 11).

Despite the numerous problems associated with alcohol, there is an enormous appetite for it and paternalistic attempts to control its use are divisive, controversial and unpopular. Opinions are often polarized, with 'nanny' killjoy moralizers on one side and the liberal open minded on the other. Nicholls (2009: 251) argues that, historically:

> The public discourse on drink has often been characterised by elements of moral panic: over-identification of problematic behaviours with 'deviant' social groups, the use of media pressure to effect policy changes, and the tendency to articulate broader social anxieties through an attack on public drunkenness.

In other words, drink, or the behaviour of certain drinkers, has been used by opponents to support stricter regulation and by supporters to back more lenient regulation. Both parties often point to the same phenomena to support their case. Folk devils – the young, working class, students, women, musicians, artists, liberals and football hooligans (visible manifestations of drunkenness) – the argument goes, have been 'created' to exaggerate a problem and propound a political agenda. On the one hand, these groups (those who drink too much) provide the evidence that alcohol is bad and more control is needed, while on the other hand their behaviour is proof that the problem is a problem for *them*. Others are able to enjoy alcohol without these negative consequences. In other words, alcohol *per se* is not the problem; rather, it is the way certain people abuse or misuse alcohol that is problematic. Currently, there is a focus in the UK and elsewhere on 'binge drinking' among the younger generation (the latest folk devils). Young men and women, including high-profile athletes, increasingly choose to get drunk in city centre bars and clubs or holiday resorts, with very visible consequences such as violence, sexual abuse, vandalism and public disorder. Such high-profile alcohol problems can detract from, and often mask, other less obvious alcohol-related issues. While the young binge drinker, beer or shot in hand, is criticized, the middle classes binging regularly on expensive red wine escape our moral gaze because they are enjoying alcohol in a civilized way and causing no obvious harm. Alcohol-related problems, however, are not confined to the young binge drinkers. Older people are increasingly facing alcohol-related health problems, but such concerns are not as newsworthy as stories about binge drinking.[3] Alcohol can be harmful in a number of ways other than intoxication, which means that a significant proportion of drinkers are potentially at risk in one way or another. Furthermore, those who do not use alcohol can be harmed directly or indirectly by those who do.

Alcohol-related harms and risk

We now know that alcohol is overwhelmingly toxic and is affecting the physical health of millions of people. According to the World Health Organization's (WHO) global status report on alcohol and health in 2014, alcohol is causally implicated in more than 200 health conditions including HIV/AIDS and tuberculosis (WHO 2014). Babor et al. (2010: 16) argue that: 'No other commodity sold for ingestion, not even tobacco, has such wide-ranging adverse physical effects'. There are 3.3 million deaths a year (5.9% of all deaths) attributable to alcohol, and 5.1% of the global burden of disease is alcohol-related. The WHO (2014: 2) suggest that although the 'consumption of alcohol and problems related to alcohol vary widely around the world, . . . the burden of disease and death remains significant in most countries'. In Australia, more than 5500 lives are lost every year as a result of alcohol and more than 157 000 people are hospitalized.[4] In the UK in 2010/2011 there were 1 168 300 alcohol-related admissions to hospitals, more than double the figure in 2002/2003.[5] According to a report by leading experts in the UK entitled 'Health first: an evidenced-based alcohol strategy for the UK', 'alcohol-related deaths in the UK have doubled from 4,023 in 1992 to 8,748 in 2011' (University of Sterling 2013: 13). In the USA, excessive alcohol consumption is responsible for the deaths of over 79 000 citizens each year (Bouchery et al. 2011). Charles Kennedy, the former leader of the Liberal Democrats parliamentary party in the UK, died recently at the age of 55 from a haemorrhage linked to alcohol abuse.[6]

Many of the conditions caused by alcohol are chronic, brought about by excessive habitual use. According to Babor et al. (2010: 15), there is clear evidence that alcohol can cause cancer of the mouth, oesophagus, larynx and pharynx, and alcohol is the main cause of liver cirrhosis. In the UK, deaths from liver disease have increased by 400% since 1970, with alcohol being the primary cause.[7] These chronic health issues were thought to affect only older drinkers, but are increasingly affecting younger drinkers. Other problems include increased risk of stroke, heart disease and brain damage. Another risk associated with alcohol is dependence or addiction. There is, perhaps unsurprisingly, a correlation between high levels of engagement in alcohol consumption by the general population and the rate of alcohol dependence within that population (Rehm and Eschmann 2002 cited Babor et al. 2010: 20). Despite this correlation, the direction of causality is unclear. 'Dependence may perpetuate heavy drinking, or heavy drinking may contribute to the developments of dependence, or these two mechanisms may operate simultaneously' (Babor et al. 2010: 20). Addiction to alcohol or other drugs is not an inevitable consequence, but is a genuine risk, particularly for those predisposed. According to Morse (2011: 176), most people who use 'potentially addicting substances do not become addicts, but between 15% and 17% do' (I will talk more about addiction in Chapter 6).

There are also acute physical harms associated with consuming excessive amounts of alcohol in one go, or binging. Binge drinking involves consuming large quantities of alcohol in a short period of time which results in intoxication (and often bad behaviour). Binge drinking and its consequences are well publicized, and, as mentioned above, policy makers and reformers are often preoccupied with it, especially on certain occasions. According to Sigman (2013: 45) this is partly because it is 'the most immediate and visible form of alcohol misuse strongly linked to anti-social behaviour, crime and accidents'. It can also lead to other serious health risks. Alcohol poisoning, acute pancreatitis or acute cardiac arrhythmias can all result from binge drinking. Fatalities can occur from episodic excessive consumption even if the binge is not characteristic of normal consumption. In other words, you can die the first time you get drunk. That acute alcohol toxicity kills is well documented. There have been countless 'rock star' deaths from alcohol binges. For example, John Bonham (drummer with Led Zeppelin, 1980), Bon Scott (lead singer with AC/DC, 1980) and Stuart Cable (former drummer with Welsh rock band Stereophonics, 2010) all died by choking on their own vomit following excessive alcohol binges. More recently, the talented singer Amy Winehouse died of alcohol poisoning at her home in July 2011 following a heavy alcohol binge. In sport, Derek Boogaard, a Canadian professional hockey player, died in 2011 as a result of an alcohol and oxycodone overdose.[8] In the USA, six people a day (mostly men) die of alcohol poisoning,[9] and more than 1800 students die each year in the USA from alcohol-related causes.[10] The Institute for Policy Research estimated that the cost of binge drinking in the UK is about £4.9 billion a year.[11]

There is a host of other harms that arise because of alcohol's psychoactive properties. It changes personality and behaviour, initially in a desirable direction. If too much is consumed, however, initial positive changes, such as relaxation, a sense of well-being and increased confidence, can quickly give way to a loss of control. Alcohol intoxication is one of the 'main causes of alcohol-related harm in the general population' (Babor et al. 2010: 16). Intoxication is associated with psychomotor impairment, slowed reaction time, impaired judgement, emotional changes and decreased sensitivity to social expectations. Alcohol's effect on judgement and inhibition leads to numerous problems. Alcohol is implicated in accidents that lead to injury and death. Falling off balconies at hotels and drowning in pools, rivers and lakes are real dangers, particularly for young people 'having a good time' with alcohol. It has long been known that driving while under the influence of alcohol is dangerous, both to the driver and other road users. As a consequence, most countries have laws forbidding driving after having consumed a specific quantity of alcohol. Significant progress has been made in reducing harms associated with driving under the influence through a combination of legislation and education. Sigman (2011) argues that both pedestrians and cyclists are also in peril when they drink alcohol. In the UK, '74% of pedestrians killed between 10 pm and 4 am were over the legal limit for drivers', and, in the USA, new year and Halloween are particularly dangerous days for pedestrians, averaging 'the highest number of walkers killed in motor-vehicle crashes and a greater proportion of on-foot victims who are "legally drunk"' (Sigman 2011: 162). In fact, Sigman (2011: 163) cites research conducted in the USA which found that drunk walking was deadlier than drunk driving (a drunk walker is eight times more likely to get killed than a drunk driver). It is a similar picture for cyclists. According to Li et al. (2001: 893), in the USA 'Elevated blood alcohol concentrations are found in about one third of fatally injured bicyclists 15 years or older'.

As we know, alcohol harms are not confined to the well-being of the drinker. Societal harms vary according to the circumstances and the culture in which drinkers live and work. They include violence, domestic violence, sexual assault and rape, vandalism, anti-social behaviour, public disorder, family problems, child neglect and abuse, financial problems, days off work and educational difficulties, among others (Babor et al. 2010). It is estimated that over the Christmas period alone hangovers cost the UK economy £260 million.[12] In Australia, over a million children are estimated to be affected by the drinking of others, and in 2006/2007 over 10 000 children were in child protection because of a carer's drinking.[13]

Of violent incidents in the UK, 53% are alcohol-related[14] and 37% of domestic violence incidents involve alcohol (University of Sterling 2013: 7). The Institute for Policy Research found that binge drinking in the UK increases the number of police officers on duty at the weekend by 30%, the number of arrests by 45% and the average number of daily injury related admissions to accident and emergency units by 8% (an extra 2504 admissions per day).[15] In Australia, in 2010, more than 70 000 citizens were victims of alcohol-related assault, 25% of whom were victims of domestic violence, and 70% of prisoners involved in violent assault had consumed alcohol before committing the offence.[16] A recent study in the UK showed that a quarter of young women put up with sexual abuse by drunken men on a night out and are not particularly surprised when it happens. Nearly a third had been 'groped'.[17]

Drinking alcohol also increases the chances of becoming a victim of more serious crime. Testa and Livingston (2009: 1349) found that binge drinking is a significant risk factor for becoming a victim of rape. In particular, the majority of rapes of female college students in the USA occurred when the victim was intoxicated. Authorities in Florida are concerned about the growing number of sexual assaults of drunk and incapable girls, often passed out (and filmed and posted on social media), by drunken revellers on Spring Break. These assaults occur in broad daylight on crowded beaches surrounded by hundreds of people. The role of alcohol is undeniable and the authorities are seeking to ban the consumption of alcohol beaches during the Spring Break period.[18] Alcohol has also been found to be the key factor in so-called 'spiked drinks' or 'drug-facilitated sexual assaults' (DFSAs). A study by Hughes et al. (2007) of patients who presented at emergency departments in the UK claiming to have their drinks spiked found that none had traces of either rohypnol or gamma-hydroxybutyrate (GHB), also known as date-rape drugs, and their symptoms were likely to be the result of excess alcohol consumption. Burgess et al. (2009: 849) argue that:

> . . . the conclusions of scientific and police investigation suggest that DFSA is in fact a very limited threat. A research-based consensus found little evidence of drink-spiking with drugs among those who suspect that it facilitated their own sexual assault; alcohol is the substance most commonly detected in the blood and urine samples of women who claim to have been victims of DFSA.

The risk to their own well-being from excessive consumption and the culpability of alcohol in their misfortune is perhaps not sufficiently recognized by drinkers and not taken seriously enough by society in general.

This use and misuse of alcohol has significant financial implications for the economy. The personal, social and economic cost of alcohol in England has been estimated at £55 billion and £7.5 billion in Scotland (University of Sterling 2013). According to the *WHO handbook for action to reduce alcohol-related harm*, the total economic cost of alcohol to the European Union (EU) was estimated to be €125 billion in 2003, equivalent to 1.3% of the EU's gross domestic product (WHO 2009). In terms of financial cost, excessive drinking in the USA totalled over $223.5 billion in 2006, of which 75% was due to binge drinking (defined as consuming 4 [women] or 5 [men] or more drinks on one occasion). The costs extend beyond front-line medical expenditure (11%) to loss in workplace productivity (72%), criminal justice costs (9%) and costs related to accidents occurring while driving under the influence of alcohol (Bouchery et al. 2011). Certain costs could not be calculated, for example, those incurred by friends and family of the excessive drinker; nevertheless, excessive drinking was estimated to cost $746 per man, woman and child in the USA in 2006. In Australia, the total estimated costs of alcohol-related problems in 2010 was $14 352 billion (20.6% criminal justice system, 11.7% health system, 42.1% Australian productivity, 25.5% traffic accidents).[19] According to Matzopolous et al. (2014), harmful use of alcohol in South Africa cost 10–12% (R 300 billion) of the country's gross domestic product in 2009. In most countries the costs of these alcohol-related harms (hospital treatment, emergency services, street cleaning, policing and so on) is unjustifiably borne by the taxpayer. In the UK, local councils are entitled to impose a levy on licensed premises to help pay for policing and cleaning, but only one city (Newcastle) is making use of it.[20]

Too many drinking too much

Some claim that the problems discussed above are caused by an 'irresponsible' minority of drinkers, but far more people are drinking too much than we might think. There are many reasons why people drink too much. Some deliberately set out to get drunk for the enjoyment or escape, or because it is 'the done thing'. Others may drink too much because they are ignorant of, or indifferent to, how much it is safe to drink. Others might be dependent on alcohol in some way. One important factor is that there is a significant difference between what most people consider to be acceptable or 'normal' drinking and the health-related advice on safe and sensible drinking levels produced by various health organizations. Although there have been clear guidelines about how much alcohol it is safe to consume for a while, these amounts are often at odds with long-established drinking cultures and practices. Advice on safe alcohol consumption is often expressed in terms of how many standard units of alcohol it is wise to drink in a day/week. A pint of beer (5.2% alcohol by volume [ABV]) is 3 units, a 175 ml glass of wine (12% ABV) is 2.1 units and a double (50 ml) measure of spirits (40% ABV) is

2 units.[21] In the UK the National Health Service (NHS) recommends that men should not regularly drink more than 3–4 units of alcohol a day and that women should not regularly (most days a week) drink more than 2–3 units a day. Drinking 1 pint of beer a day will take a man up to his weekly limit. The Royal College of Psychiatrists say that 6 units for women and 8 units for men over a short period of time constitute a binge.[22] This equates to just over 2 pints (approximately 1000 ml) of 5% ABV beer or fewer than three (175 ml) glasses of wine for women, and fewer than 3 pints of 5% ABV beer or under four (175 ml) glasses of wine for men. There are some products (strong lager) where drinking one can or bottle exceeds the recommended units.

Data from numerous sources seems to support the idea that people either do not know how much they should be drinking, or are indifferent to the guidelines. In the UK, in 2010, 35% of men and 28% of women drank more than the government recommended daily units of alcohol on at least one day prior to interview, and 19% of men and 12% of women reported drinking twice the recommended daily intake on at least one day prior to interview. There is an enduring pattern of men drinking more than women and young people drinking more than older people. In 2010, 6% of men reported drinking over double the recommended levels (over 50 units a week on average) and 3% of women reported drinking over 35 units in an average week.[23] In 2010/2011, 17% of men and 10% of women over the age of 16 reported drinking on 5 or more days in the week prior to interview, and 9% of men and 5% of women reported drinking every day.[24] There is a similar picture in the USA where 15% adults reported binge drinking.[25] In Canada, between 4 and 5 million people engage in high-risk drinking, and Canadians drink 50% more than the global average (WHO 2014). Generally speaking, men are drinking more and more often than women. In the Republic of Ireland, 54% of 18–75 year olds were classified as harmful drinkers in 2013 and one in 14 met the criteria for dependent drinking.[26]

These disturbing figures are likely to underestimate the true picture. According to Babor et al. (2010: 23), although surveys provide important data about drinking patterns, they tend to underestimate consumption by 30–70%. Boniface and Shelton (2013: 1076) suggest that international reported alcohol consumption equates to between 40 and 60% of total alcohol sales. In other words, much more alcohol is sold than we admit to drinking. Using data from Her Majesty's Revenue and Customs (HMRC) in the UK, Boniface and Shelton (2013) compared the amount sold with figures from two self-reporting alcohol consumption surveys conducted in 2008.[27] Their results showed that almost half of the alcohol sold was not accounted for in the self-reporting figures. The results confirm concerns surrounding the reliability of self-reported surveys of alcohol consumption, but more importantly paint a more accurate picture of the extent of alcohol consumption in the UK. Taking account of the under-reporting, Boniface and Shelton (2013) estimate that over a third of UK adults are drinking above weekly guidelines and over three quarters drank above the recommended daily guidelines once in the week prior to the survey. The message from the data is unequivocal. Too many people are drinking too much alcohol too often.

Harm reduction and alcohol policy

Unsurprisingly, given the disease burden of alcohol misuse, many national and international organizations, such as the WHO, the UK NHS and the National Institute on Alcohol Abuse and Alcoholism in the USA, are committed to reducing harm caused by alcohol. There is a clear consensus, at least among health organizations, that there needs to be a reduction in the amount of global alcohol consumed in order to reduce harms. In particular, the WHO (2014: vii) concludes that:

> In the light of a growing population worldwide and the predicted increase in alcohol consumption in the world, the alcohol attributable disease burden as well as the social and economic burden may increase further unless effective prevention policies and measures based on the best available evidence are implemented worldwide.

Policies aimed at curtailing supply and/or reducing demand are unwelcome by consumers and producers. They are seen as anti-liberal and paternalistic. Moreover, the production and consumption of alcohol is lucrative in terms of profits and tax revenue and the industry creates jobs. There is, therefore, some reluctance on the part of governments to regulate the industry too tightly. Like other economically powerful industries whose products might be harmful, breweries and distilleries seem able to influence government policy in their favour. They push the view that education rather than regulation is the answer to any problems caused by drink.

In the UK, there is a particularly powerful alcohol lobby influencing government policy. Despite the known risks of alcohol consumption and the growing problem of anti-social drinking, the then Labour government took the counter-intuitive (and with hindsight, blatantly misguided) decision to further relax licensing laws in 2005, allowing premises to sell alcohol 24 hours a day. Incomprehensibly, the rationale was a harm-reduction one. It was expected that consumers would slow down their drinking, thus avoiding intoxication. It was thought that consumers would adopt a more 'Mediterranean' approach to drinking; in other words, drinking more slowly and in a more 'civilized' way. But France, the exemplar of civilized alcohol consumption, is itself looking to legislate to reduce binge drinking.[28] Far from reducing harms, these changes in the law are being blamed for the growth in alcohol-related crime and disorder in the UK.[29] A number of towns and cities have a burgeoning weekend night-time economy geared around supplying alcohol and 'good times' to revellers who visit in their thousands. The latest figures from the UK government show that there are 208 areas in the UK saturated with public houses and nightclubs, an increase of 30% in just 2 years. The alcohol-fuelled disorder in these areas, also known as 'stress areas', is so serious that no further drinking establishments will be granted a licence.[20] Consequently, other harm-reduction measures are required to mitigate the surge in problems. There has been an increase in law enforcement resources allocated to monitor city centres in an attempt to deter and manage disorder. Most city centres have a visible police presence, particularly in known trouble spots. Plastic glasses are used in certain high-risk establishments to minimize the risks of facial injuries, some city centre roads have been pedestrianized to allow drunken revellers more room to avoid each other and taxi ranks have introduced stewards to minimize the threat of disorder as revellers argue over cabs.[30] Research has also shown that a higher density of outlets selling alcohol is associated with intimate partner violence (Kearns et al. 2015).

According to Moore and Heikkinen (2013), another significant consequence of mass city centre drinking are the implications for the ambulance service and hospitals in dealing with alcohol-related injuries. They argue that the consequence of the inevitable increase in alcohol-related emergency admission is that 'staff may need to prioritize the severely intoxicated leaving perhaps more legitimate patients waiting' (Moore and Heikkinen 2013: 710). Another issue facing hospital staff is the physical and verbal abuse they face at the hands of both the drunken patient and friends and family members attending the accident and emergency departments late at night.[31] In the city of Cardiff they have sought to address this problem by introducing what might be called a 'drunk tank' in the form of a temporary 'field hospital' in the city centre during certain events. The temporary facility is staffed by medics and means that the intoxicated injured are not taken to the main hospital (unless of course their injuries require it). The problems are exacerbated during certain celebratory events such as sporting occasions, New Year's Eve and so on. One such event is 'Black Friday', the last Friday before Christmas, which sees thousands of office workers leave work early to drink in the city centre.[32] The consequences are often 'black' as the press reported: 'The makeshift medical centre at the Millennium Stadium [the city's 75 000-capacity sporting arena] in Cardiff dealt with scores of drunken revellers as "black Friday" hit the Welsh capital' (Smith 2011). Such strategies aimed at minimizing harms associated with excessive drinking might be effective inasmuch as injuries are treated more quickly, and the emergency room at the hospital is not inundated with injured drunks.

Another set of initiatives to ameliorate the harms associated with the city centre binge-drinking culture in the UK is mentioned by Sigman (2011). In London, Camden Council is tackling the anti-social consequences by handing out free flip-flops, tea, biscuits and lollipops on Friday and Saturday nights. Flip-flops prevent women damaging their feet when they remove their high heels and the biscuits and lollipops make people less aggressive. Such measures may provide some benefit (reduction in certain harms, injuries and criminal offences), but Sigman (2011) argues that these measures (and I would add, many of the other measures mentioned) serve to enable, condone and normalize the behaviour. They are a sticking plaster to cover the real issue of customers drinking too much and policies that allow the almost unregulated supply of alcohol. City centres have become no-go areas for non-drinkers and families. Moore and Heikkinen (2013: 710) argue that although dealing in the most effective way with medical and criminal outcomes such as designated medical facilities, targeted policing and the like is crucial, a '. . . better understanding of why a significant proportion of drinkers exceed safe limits and what might be done to challenge this . . .' is needed. The choice of going to town centre bars and clubs to drink, particularly at the weekend, remains a popular one for young adults in most Western countries. Nutt (2012: 67) observes that: 'In recent years, a new trend has emerged among young people in the UK, of deliberately trying to get so intoxicated, usually on alcohol, that they have no memory of getting "wasted" or "ended"'. This often means pre-loading on cheap alcohol before going out. Of course, getting drunk is not restricted to town centres; other venues such as popular holiday resorts also have significant problems. Recent figures by the Civil Aviation Authority, for example, show that there has been a significant rise in alcohol-related disruptive behaviour on flights.[33]

There may be many reasons why this behaviour is common, but there is a broad consensus (outside the alcohol industry) that a significant part of the problem is the availability of cheap alcohol. In the UK, relative to income levels, alcohol is three times cheaper than it was in the 1950s, and consumption has continued to climb since then. Moreover, it is easier than ever before to buy alcohol from a range of outlets at any time of the day or night. Despite the increase in supply and relative reduction in price, there has been a refusal to make the basic economic connection between the increase in demand and consumption. As mentioned, UK government policy has seen a relaxation of licensing laws. To date, there has been a reluctance on the part of the UK government to implement stronger controls on sales and pricing, favouring instead an educational campaign, including heavy-hitting TV advertisements, aimed at warning people about the dangers of excessive consumption. The resistance to legislation and a focus on education (to promote sensible choice) is coupled with, or driven by, the powerful influence of the alcohol industry. Nutt (2012) argues that the alcohol industry is preoccupied with protecting the public image of its product despite the growing evidence of the harms it causes.

According to the European Centre for Monitoring Alcohol Marketing's publication, *The seven key messages of the alcohol industry*, the industry seeks to perpetuate the following about its product.

1   Consuming alcohol is normal, common, healthy and very responsible.
2   The damage done by alcohol is caused by a small group of deviants who cannot handle alcohol.
3   Normal adult non-drinkers do not, in fact, exist.
4   Ignore the fact that alcohol is a harmful and addictive chemical substance (ethanol) for the body.
5   Alcohol problems can only be solved when all parties work together.
6   Alcohol marketing is not harmful. It is simply intended to assist the consumer in selecting a certain product or brand.
7   Education about responsible use is the best method to protect society from alcohol problems (European Centre for Monitoring Alcohol Marketing 2011).

Nutt (2012) believes that these messages range from distortions of the truth to outright lies. They work to normalize alcohol use and, despite the industry's claims to the contrary, a substantial profit is made by the misuse of alcohol. In fact,

Nutt (2012: 101) argues that if all drinking above recommended levels in the UK ceased there would be a drop of 40% in consumption, equating to a £13 billion loss of revenue for alcohol companies. Alcohol misuse is self-evidently profitable for alcohol companies.

These concerns about government involvement with the alcohol industry in the UK are shared by some inside the government itself. Nutt (2012: 94) reports that concerns were raised by the House of Commons 2010 Health Committee's report when it expressed the following:

> We are concerned that Government policies are much closer to, and too influenced by those of the drinks industry and the supermarkets than those of expert health professionals such as the Royal College of Physicians or the CMO [Chief Medical Officer].

Furthermore, Richard Gartside, the director of the UK's Centre for Crime and Justice Studies, was very critical of the UK government's failure to take sufficient notice of the scientific evidence on alcohol-related harms, and was 'dismayed that the home secretary appears to believe that political calculation trumps honest and informed scientific opinion'.[34]

The WHO (2014) have argued that the range of harms provide a concrete rationale for developing national and international alcohol policy aimed at minimizing alcohol-related harms. The UK government agree that alcohol consumption needs to be brought under control, but disagree about the most effective means. Research shows (despite the protestations of the alcohol industry among others) that:

> ... the use of taxation to regulate the demand for alcoholic beverages, restricting their availability and implementing bans of alcohol advertising – are the 'best buys' in reduction the harmful use of alcohol . . . (WHO 2014: 19).

According to Nutt (2012: 105): 'Evidence from across the world shows that the price of alcohol determines use for almost everyone, with the possible exception of severely dependent drinkers'. According to Sigman (2011: 235): 'It is estimated that a minimum price 50p [pence] per unit would save over 3000 lives per year, and a minimum price of 40p, 1100 lives' in the UK. In the USA, Wagenaar et al. (2010) suggested that doubling the tax on alcohol would reduce alcohol-related mortality by about 35% and road deaths by about 11%. Wagenaar et al. (2015) also found that the increase in alcohol tax in the state of Illinois in 2009 led to a 26% fall in fatal car accidents involving alcohol. There is growing pressure in the UK for an increase in alcohol price and the House of Commons Health Committee strongly recommends that the government introduce minimum pricing, but such recommendations have been resisted.[35] Raising the price of alcohol would be a vote loser among those who feel their pockets would be affected. Opponents of such regulation argue that such measures would not be needed if people drank responsibly and that responsible drinkers will be punished unnecessarily. The reality is that a minimum price of 40p per unit would cost a genuine moderate drinker an extra 11p a week.

Controlling the marketing and promotion of alcohol is also an important strategy in harm reduction. Nutt (2012:106) believes that: 'All alcohol advertising should be banned, and drinks containing alcohol should have warning notices similar to those on cigarette packets'. This of course would have serious implications for sport given its close commercial alliance with alcohol companies. In most countries there are some rules about how and when alcohol can be advertised but the budget spent on marketing far outstrips the budget for education. There is also evidence to support the eradication of cheap drink offers, below-cost sales (such as supermarket promotions) and bringing an end to government subsidies for bars such as university student unions. Other strategies of reducing alcohol consumption might involve banning events and organizations which offer cheap drink and/or explicitly promote binge drinking. In the UK there is a nationwide student event called Carnage.[36] It is essentially an organized pub crawl for students hosted in cities across the UK, and has unsurprisingly come in for severe criticism, not least when a student participating in an event was photographed urinating on a war memorial in the city of Sheffield.[37] My own university's (Cardiff Metropolitan University) student union has had a long tradition of a bi-annual end-of-term celebration called 'drink the bar dry'. The name clearly implies that heavy drinking is the order of the day. Recently the name has been changed because a neighbouring university's (Cardiff University) student union was criticized in the local press for using the title.[38] These types of excessive drinking event, especially given the target audience are young people (see below), are particularly problematic and should be discouraged.

Perhaps the clearest indication of the alcohol industry's hegemony in the UK is to be found in the organization primarily responsible for delivering the education message, namely Drinkaware. The Drinkaware Trust is an independent charitable trust whose aim is to promote sensible drinking. Citizens in the UK will be familiar with their efforts in the context of alcohol advertisements on television or in cinemas where an inconspicuous tagline appears at the end of a colourful advertisement extolling the virtues of a particular brand. The tagline reads 'please drink responsibly'. According to Sigman (2011), Drinkaware is almost entirely funded by the alcohol industry. Some £2.2 million of the £2.6 million received in donations by Drinkaware in 2008 came from the Portman Group.[39] The Portman Group comprises the nine biggest drinks companies in the UK including Carlsberg UK, Heineken UK and Molson Coors Brewing Company UK. In Sigman's (2011: 223) words, this amounts to 'leaving a vital area of health education in the hands of the poachers, as opposed to the game keepers'. It is clear that not only is it in the interest of these companies to keep people drinking, but to recruit new drinkers. The situation is farcical and unsurprisingly the WHO (2014: 24) is unequivocal in its assessment: '. . . the alcohol industry has no role in the formulation of alcohol policies'. Katherine Brown, director of the Institute for Alcohol Studies, based in London, is clear about the conflict of interest, arguing that 'you have an industry whose primary motive is to look after the profits of its shareholders . . . versus the public health objective that will cut its profits'.[40] McCambridge et al. (2014: 3) are particularly critical of the way the alcohol industry influences governments in the UK and Australia which leads to bad policies. They argue that the industry is using their power to set the agenda and shape policy: 'The alcohol industry's favoured definition of harm reduction actually entails harm promotion, however well-constructed the smokescreen of self-serving ideas'. In the USA, there is also concern about industry self-regulation and industry-led 'drink responsibly' campaigns which only serve to protect profits and 'allow alcohol producers to blame youth, parents, and anyone but their own corporate actions for the staggering health and economic harm from alcohol products, while making alcohol companies look socially responsible'.[41]

Double standards

It is interesting and insightful to compare the general attitude towards alcohol, the reluctance to legislate more strongly in relation to alcohol with the attitudes and laws pertaining to other drugs. In 2009, Professor Nutt was sacked from his post as advisor to the UK government on drugs for claiming that alcohol was more dangerous than certain illegal drugs such as ecstasy (a view based on research detailed below). His assessment of the situation was not welcomed by the UK government because it potentially undermined the existing government policies which involve a tough stance on drugs (which sees the criminalization of use and/ or possession of certain drugs such as ecstasy and cannabis) and a comparatively liberal alcohol policy.[42] In his book, *Drugs without the hot air*, Nutt (2012) opens a chapter entitled 'If alcohol were discovered today, would it be legal?', with the following vignette:

> A TERRIFYING new 'legal high' has hit our streets. Methylcarbonol, known by the street name 'wiz', is a clear liquid that causes cancers, liver problems, and brain disease, and is more toxic than ecstasy and cocaine. Addiction can occur after just one drink, and addicts will go to any lengths to get their next fix – even letting their kids go hungry or beating up their partners to obtain money. Casual users can go into blind RAGES when they're high and police have reported a huge increase in crime where the drug is being used. Worst of all, drinks companies are adding 'wiz' to fizzy drinks and advertising them to kids like they're plain Coca-Cola. Two or three teenagers die from it EVERY WEEK overdosing on a binge, and another TEN from having accidents caused by reckless driving. 'Wiz' is a public menace – when will the Home Secretary make this dangerous substance Class A?

Clearly, the vignette refers to alcohol and is constructed to be deliberately provocative. However, the claims made about 'wiz' are based on scientific evidence about the effects of alcohol. Is it reasonable to claim, however, that alcohol is more dangerous than other drugs? Is the comparison of alcohol (a legal drug) with heroin (an illegal drug with a global reputation for severe harm) a reasonable one? Nutt et al. (2010) put together a panel of experts to construct a matrix of drug- and alcohol-related harms with the aim of providing transparent information about how much harm is caused by alcohol and other drugs in the UK. They assessed the relative harms associated with 20 drugs including alcohol, heroin, cocaine, crack cocaine and cannabis. Each drug was scored out of 100 on 16 criteria, nine relating to harm to the individual (for example, harm caused by the drug directly such as alcohol-related cirrhosis) and seven relating to harms caused to others (for example, injury resulting in alcohol-related violence). As might be expected, heroin, crack cocaine and metamfetamine scored highest in relation to harm to self, but alcohol scored higher than both heroin and crack cocaine in relation to harm to others. When the scores were combined, alcohol came out very badly. 'Overall, alcohol was the most harmful drug (overall harm score 72), with heroin (55) and crack cocaine (54) in second and third places' (Nutt et al. 2010: 1558). The findings are unpalatable because they challenge society's attitudes towards alcohol, not least because certain demonized class A drugs like ecstasy were found to be relatively harmless. The findings, or perhaps the way they were reported in the UK media, led to Professor Nutt's dismissal.

For a host of legal, sociopolitical and historical reasons, the dominant attitude towards drugs and alcohol are very different. In the UK, over the last decade there have been a number of 'legal highs' such as mephedrone ('meow meow'), which were criminalized as a consequence of their alleged role in the deaths of youngsters. Nutt (2012: 114) argues that, according to toxicology reports, neither of the two deaths attributed to mephedrone that hit the headlines in the UK in 2010 were attributable to the substance. Rather, the two young men died from a lethal combination of alcohol and methadone (both legally available). Nevertheless, the deaths were connected to mephedrone in the media at the time, resulting in a 'moral panic' and calls for its criminalization. The UK government duly obliged, based on little or no evidence of its harmful effects. The Conservative government, elected in 2015, promised to introduce a new bill that would make the sale of all psychoactive substances illegal apart from alcohol, tobacco and caffeine.[43] There is also a particular fear of ecstasy in the UK after the well-publicized death of a young girl (Leah Betts) in 1995 after taking two ecstasy tablets. According to Nutt (2012), her death was the result of water intoxication (hyponatraemia). Ecstasy-related deaths have reduced following a public information campaign advising people how much water to drink. The seemingly unjustified scaremongering about date-rape drugs when it appears that too much alcohol is mostly to blame for rendering victims vulnerable is further evidence of the disproportionate fear of drugs in comparison with alcohol. Some drugs do pose a significant risk, but, despite high-profile deaths, ecstasy and speed continue to be used routinely by young people without the widespread apocalyptic consequences which befell a very small minority of consumers, but which routinely befall drinkers.

Starting young

Given the problems associated with alcohol, a key concern is the extent young people are affected by it. Most countries restrict the supply of alcohol to children or people under a certain age, although the particular age varies from country to country. In the UK, licensed premises are not permitted to sell alcohol to people under the age of 18, and in most states in the USA you have to be over 21 years of age. In the UK, however, it is legal for parents to give their children alcohol at home from the age of 5, children can go into certain public houses but cannot drink alcohol and at 16 years of age can drink (but not buy) alcohol in public houses with a meal. In Finland it is a crime for parents to supply their children with alcohol.[44] According to Sigman (2013: 42): 'Europeans start drinking long before they reach adulthood' and nowhere is the normalization of alcohol (in comparison with other drugs) more obvious, risky and inconsistent than in the context of children and young people. Many parents believe that the responsible thing to do is to initiate their children into alcohol believing that early experience will be protective from later misuse. Alcohol, however, is even more toxic to children than to adults and they face additional risks from consuming alcohol. Research shows that:

> ... the developing adolescent brain may be particularly susceptible to long-term negative consequences from alcohol use. Recent studies show that alcohol consumption has the potential to trigger long-term biological changes that may have detrimental effects on the developing adolescent brain, including neurocognitive impairment.[45]

Even small amounts of alcohol change the growing brains of children. According to Sigman (2011: 84): 'These alcohol-related changes are linked directly to our children's intellect, personality, mental and physical health'.[46] All the evidence points towards delaying the age at which people start to drink and 'in an ideal world, young people should not consume any alcohol – including having a drink with parents at home – until they have reached the age of 24.5 years' (Sigman 2013: 61). The USA is ahead of the UK (and many other countries) in terms of alcohol policy in this regard. The USA government has insisted that all states raise the legal drinking age to 21 years of age and many states do not let those under 21 years of age drink anywhere, including at home (Sigman 2011). Gruenewald (2011: 249) questions why any government would set a minimum legal drinking age below 21 years. There are, of course, other considerations in setting the minimum legal drinking age such as tax revenue, but the evidence points in a different direction to many of our cultural habits and attitudes in relation to drink. In light of the evidence, Sigman (2013) argues that the introduction of alcohol by parents to children at a young age is seriously misguided. 'It is a fundamental misconception such practices cultivate 'responsible drinking' in teenagers' (Sigman 2013: 45). Evidence shows that: 'The early introduction to an addictive substance leads to a greater likelihood of addiction' (Sigman 2013: 45). In the UK, the Chief Medical

Officer's report 'Guidance on the consumption of alcohol by young people' (Department of Health 2009) offers unequivocal advice for parents; namely that an alcohol-free childhood is the best option. Sellman et al. (2010: 772) argue that giving children alcohol to remove the taboo and lessen the 'big deal' of alcohol is not a good idea; 'evidence points in the opposite direction, that normalization of alcohol increases the risk of harm'. In England, school pupils are more likely to have drunk alcohol if someone they live with did and pupils who felt that their families would not want them to drink are less likely to do so.

> 87% of pupils who felt that their parents would disapprove had never drank alcohol compared with 28% of those who thought that their parents wouldn't mind as long as they didn't drink too much (Fuller 2012: 2).

A longitudinal study by Jackson et al. (2015) found that students who had sipped alcohol (given a taste by their parents) by the time they had reached sixth grade (11–12 years old) were five times more likely to have consumed a full drink, and four times more likely to have binged or been drunk, by the time they got to high school than their peers.

Statistics on drinking prevalence among children are likely to suffer from similar reliability issues as discussed above, nevertheless they point to problems with underage drinking. White and Jackson (2004/2005: 183) identify alcohol as a means used by emerging adults to 'seek out altered states of consciousness'. It is one of the substances that adolescents consume in their sensation-seeking behaviour (White and Jackson 2004/2005: 186). According to Fuller (2012), in 2012, 43% of all 11–15 year olds in England had drank alcohol at least once that year. The figure for 15-year-old children was 74%. Ten per cent of pupils had drank alcohol in the preceding week (down from 25% in 2003). Those who had drank had consumed an average of 12.5 units and 50% of children who had drank in the preceding month had been drunk (61% deliberately, 39% not deliberately). In the USA, two out of five 15 year olds have drank alcohol, 24.3% of 12–20 year olds had drank alcohol in the past month, 15% of this age group were binge drinkers (5.9 million people) and 4.3% were heavy drinkers. It is estimated that 3.4% of 12–17 year olds had an alcohol-use disorder (855 000) with 76 000 adolescents receiving treatment for their drinking at a rehabilitation centre.[47] It is estimated that the cost to the USA economy of underage drinking in 2013 ran to $56.9 billion, which includes an estimated $36.9 billion in what they call pain and suffering costs. Even without these costs, the tangible costs of medical care, criminal justice, property damage and loss of work came to $20.01 billion (youth violence alone cost $32 million).[48] Young people are at a greater risk from alcohol problems because the alcohol they drink is more likely to be consumed as a binge; they also are less risk-averse and may engage in more reckless behaviour when drunk (WHO 2014). It seems that 'alcopops', alcoholic drinks that are flavoured or sweetened and are more palatable to young people, and some would argue designed and aimed at the young drinker's market, are of particular concern. According to Albers et al. (2015), underage drinkers who drink alcopops exclusively are more likely to engage in binge drinking and suffer from alcohol-related injuries. There are some signs that the pattern of alcohol consumption in the UK is changing and that more people, especially young people, are abstaining from alcohol altogether, and that fewer are drinking as often or as much. Nevertheless, the total amount of alcohol sold in the UK is enough to take every consumer over the recommended guidelines.[49]

Summary

Alcohol is a potentially dangerous psychoactive drug, especially when misused. For many, risky drinking is actually normal drinking. Alcohol use is considered the norm; its misuse is tolerated (whereas drug misuse is demonized) and in some subcultures encouraged or at least tacitly condoned. Of particular concern is the way children and young people are exposed to a culture of drinking and for some grow up being encouraged to drink. In the next chapter I discuss ways in which sport has, and continues to play, a role in the normalization of alcohol consumption.

Notes

1 See Nicholls (2009) for an extended history of alcohol in England.
2 http://en.wikipedia.org/wiki/Volstead_Act (accessed 10/04/2015).
3 http://www.bbc.co.uk/news/uk-wales-26143702 (accessed 10/04/2015).
4 http://www.fare.org.au/wp-content/uploads/2015/02/01-ALCOHOLS-IMPACT-ON-CHILDREN-AND-FAMILIES-web.pdf (accessed 1/05/2015).
5 http://www.hscic.gov.uk/catalogue/PUB06166/alco-eng-2012-rep.pdf (accessed 10/04/2015).
6 http://www.bbc.co.uk/news/uk-politics-33025795 (accessed 6/07/2015).
7 http://www.thelancet.com/commissions/crisis-of-liver-disease-in-the-UK (accessed 5/05/2015).
8 http://en.wikipedia.org/wiki/Derek_Boogaard#Death (accessed 10/04/2014).
9 http://www.cdc.gov/vitalsigns/alcohol-poisoning-deaths/index.html (accessed 1/05/2015).
10 http://www.nytimes.com/2014/12/15/us/why-colleges-havent-stopped-binge-drinking.html?_r=3 (accessed 1/05/2015).
11 http://www.bath.ac.uk/ipr/pdf/policy-briefs/cost-of-binge-drinking.pdf (accessed 29/04/2015).
12 http://www.bbc.com/capital/story/20150102-the-real-cost-of-hangovers (accessed 1/05/2015).
13 http://www.fare.org.au/hto2015/ (accessed 5/05/2015).
14 http://www.alcoholpolicy.net/2015/02/53-of-violent-incidents-alcohol-related-british-crime-survey-201314.html (accessed 1/05/2015).
15 http://www.bath.ac.uk/ipr/pdf/policy-briefs/cost-of-binge-drinking.pdf (accessed 29/04/2015).
16 http://www.alcohol.sa.gov.au/site/page.cfm?u=489 (accessed 11/04/2013).
17 http://www.telegraph.co.uk/women/womens-life/11087929/Quarter-of-young-women-put-up-with-sexual-abuse-on-a-night-out.html (accessed 5/05/2015).
18 http://edition.cnn.com/2015/04/15/us/florida-panama-city-beach-spring-break/index.html (accessed 30/04/2015).
19 http://www.aic.gov.au/publications/current%20series/tandi/441-460/tandi454.html (accessed 18/04/2013).

20 http://www.telegraph.co.uk/news/uknews/law-and-order/11308576/Alcohol-saturated-areas-soar-as-measures-fail-to-dilute-late-night-drinking-culture.html (accessed 1/05/2015).
21 http://www.nhs.uk/Livewell/alcohol/Pages/alcohol-units.aspx (accessed 10/04/2015).
22 http://www.rcpsych.ac.uk/healthadvice/problemsdisorders/alcoholourfavouritedrug.aspx (accessed 23/07/2014).
23 http://www.hscic.gov.uk/searchcatalogue?productid=7172&q=alcohol&sort=Relevance&size=10&page=1#top (accessed 11/04/2013).
24 http://www.hscic.gov.uk/catalogue/PUB06166/alco-eng-2012-rep.pdf (accessed 10/04/2015).
25 http://www.cdc.gov/alcohol/fact-sheets/alcohol-use.htm (accessed 10/04/2015).
26 http://www.hrb.ie/index.php?id=1000&tx_ttnews[tt_news]=535 (accessed 5/05/2015).
27 The General Lifestyle Survey sample, 12 490 adults, and the Health Survey for England sample, 9608 adults.
28 http://www.washingtonpost.com/blogs/worldviews/wp/2014/10/16/france-where-children-sip-wine-wants-to-end-binge-drinking/ (accessed 5/05/2015).
29 http://www.telegraph.co.uk/news/uknews/law-and-order/10543625/Huge-increase-in-towns-blighted-by-alcohol-trouble-since-drink-laws-relaxed.html (accessed 20/07/2014).
30 In particular, see the work of the Violence and Society Research Group at Cardiff University who have successfully contributed to declining alcohol-related violence in Cardiff, UK. http://www.cardiff.ac.uk/dentl/research/themes/appliedclinicalresearch/violenceandsociety/index.html (accessed 10/04/2015).
31 http://news.sky.com/story/1398616/action-urged-to-stop-drunks-abusing-nhs-staff (accessed 5/05/2015).
32 This 'Black Friday' is unconnected to the sales events at retailers in the lead up to Christmas which goes by the same name.
33 http://rt.com/uk/233455-caa-alcohol-flights-incidents/ (accessed 1/05/2014).
34 http://www.guardian.co.uk/politics/2009/oct/30/drugs-adviser-david-nutt-sacked (accessed 11/04/2013).
35 http://www.bbc.co.uk/news/uk-politics-23346532 (accessed 10/04/2015).
36 http://www.carnageuk.com/ (accessed 10/04/2015).
37 http://www.telegraph.co.uk/news/uknews/crime/6660489/Student-Philip-Laing-who-urinated-on-war-memorial-avoids-jail.html (accessed 10/04/2015).
38 http://www.walesonline.co.uk/news/local-news/the-lash-drink-bar-dry-2506118 (accessed 10/04/2015).
39 http://www.publications.parliament.uk/pa/cm200910/cmselect/cmhealth/151/151we17.htm (accessed 10/04/2015).
40 http://www.independent.ie/life/health-wellbeing/under-the-influence/expert-slams-drinks-industry-health-campaigns-31161919.html (accessed 29/04/2015).
41 https://alcoholjustice.org/watchdogging/in-the-doghouse (accessed 30/04/2015).
42 http://www.guardian.co.uk/politics/2009/oct/30/drugs-adviser-david-nutt-sacked (accessed 10/04/2013).
43 http://www.bbc.co.uk/news/uk-32926504 (accessed 6/07/2015).
44 http://yle.fi/uutiset/its_a_crime_to_supply_alcohol_to_a_minor_-_even_your_own_child/7957439 (accessed 5/05/2015).
45 The Surgeon General's call to action to prevent and reduce underage drinking. 2007, pp. v–vi. http://www.ncbi.nlm.nih.gov/books/NBK44360/ (accessed 10/04/2015).
46 See Sigman (2013) for an overview of the research detailing the extent of alcohol-related brain changes and their consequence for children.
47 http://www.niaaa.nih.gov/alcohol-health/overview-alcohol-consumption/alcohol-facts-and-statistics (accessed 10/04/2015).
48 http://www.udetc.org/UnderageDrinkingCosts.asp (accessed 29/04/2015).
49 http://www.telegraph.co.uk/news/health/news/11411081/Teetotalism-on-the-march-as-young-turn-their-back-on-drink.html (accessed 1/05/2015).

References

Albers, A.B., et al., 2015. Flavored alcoholic beverage use, risky drinking behaviors, and adverse outcomes among underage drinkers: results from the ABRAND study. *American Journal of Public Health*, 105(4), 810–815.

Babor, T., et al., 2010. *Alcohol: no ordinary commodity—research and public policy*, 2nd edn. Oxford: Oxford University Press.

Boniface, S. and Shelton, N., 2013. How is alcohol consumption affected if we account for under-reporting? A hypothetical scenario. *European Journal of Public Health*, 23(6), 1076–1081.

Bouchery, E.E., et al., 2011. Economic costs of excessive alcohol consumption in the U.S., 2006. *American Journal of Preventive Medicine*, 41(5), 516–524.

Burgess, A., Donavan, P. and Moore, S.E.H., 2009. Embodying uncertainty? Understanding heightened risk perception of drink "spiking". *British Journal of Criminology*, 49, 848–862.

Davenport-Hines, R., 2002. *The pursuit of oblivion: a social history of drugs*. London: Phoenix.

Department of Health, 2009. Guidance on the consumption of alcohol by children and young people. http://www.cph.org.uk/wp-content/uploads/2013/09/Guidance-on-the-consumption-of-alcohol-by-children-and-young-people.pdf (accessed 6/07/2015).

European Centre for Monitoring Alcohol Marketing, 2011. *The seven key messages of the alcohol industry*. http://www.iogt.org/wp-content/uploads/2011/07/Seven_key_messages1.pdf (accessed 10/04/2015).

Flanagan, O., 2011. What is it like to be an addict? In: J. Poland and G. Graham, eds. *Addiction and responsibility*. Cambridge, MA: MIT Press, 269–292.

Flanagan, O. 2013. Phenomenal authority: the epistemic authority of alcoholics anonymous. In: N. Levy, ed. *Addiction and self-control: perspectives from philosophy, psychology and neuroscience*. Oxford: Oxford University Press 67–93.

Fuller, E. (ed.), 2012. *Smoking, drinking and drug use among young people in England in 2012*. Leeds: Health and Social Care Information Centre (HSCIC).

Gruenewald, P.J., 2011. Regulating availability: how access to alcohol affects drinking and problems in youth and adults. *Alcohol Research and Health*, 34(2), 248–256.

Hughes, H., et al., 2007. A study of patients presenting to an emergency department having had a "spiked drink". *Emergency Medicine Journal*, 24, 89–91.

Jackson, K.M., et al., 2015. The prospective association between sipping alcohol by the sixth grade and later substance use. *Journal of Studies on Alcohol and Drugs*, 76(2), 212–221.

Kearns, M.C., Reidy, D.E. and Valle, L.A., 2015. The role of alcohol policies in preventing intimate partner violence: a review of the literature. *Journal of Studies on Alcohol and Drugs*, 76(1), 21–30.

Li, G., et al., 2001. Use of alcohol as a risk factor for bicycling injury. *Journal of the American Medical Association*, 285(7), 893–896.

Matzopoulos, R.G., et al., 2014. The cost of harmful alcohol use in South Africa. *South African Medical Journal*, 104(2), 127–132.

McCambridge, J., et al., 2014. Alcohol harm reduction: corporate capture of a key concept. *PLoS Medicine*, 11(12). doi: 10.1371/journal.pmed.1001767.

Moore, S.C. and Heikkinen, M., 2013. Commentary on Lloyd et al. (2013): secondary harms and opportunities for moderation, *Addiction*, 108, 710–711.

Morse, S.J., 2011. Addiction and criminal responsibility. In: J. Poland and G. Graham, eds. *Addiction and responsibility*, Cambridge, MA: MIT Press, 159–199.

Nicholls, J., 2009. *The politics of alcohol: a history of the drink question in England.* Manchester: Manchester University Press.

Nutt, D., 2012. *Drugs without the hot air: minimising the harms of legal and illegal drugs.* Cambridge: UIT Cambridge.

Nutt, D.J., King, L.A. and Phillips, L.D., 2010. Drug harms in the UK: a multicriteria decision analysis. *Lancet*, 376, 1558–1565.

Pritchard, I., 2006. *Leisure and national identity in the south Wales coalfield 1830–1914.* Thesis (PhD). Cardiff Metropolitan University.

Sellman, J.D., Connor, J.L. and Joyce, P.R., 2010. How to reduce alcohol-related problems in adolescents: what can parents do and what can the Government do? *Australian and New Zealand Journal of Psychiatry*, 44, 771–773.

Sigman, A., 2011. *Alcohol nation: how to protect our children from today's drinking culture.* London: Piatkus.

Sigman, A., 2013. Preventing alcohol use disorders among children and adolescents in the EU. In: *European Parliament working group on the quality of childhood. Improving the quality of childhood in Europe, Volume 4.* http://www.ecswe.net/downloads/publications/QOC-V4/QOC13-Chapter1-Sigman.pdf (accessed 6/07/2015).

Smith, A., 2011. Field hospital set up for Cardiff's 'black Friday' revellers. *The Telegraph.* http://www.telegraph.co.uk/topics/christmas/8962991/Field-hospital-set-up-for-Cardiffs-black-Friday-revellers.html (accessed 17/12/2012).

Testa, M. and Livingston, J.L., 2009. Alcohol consumption and women's vulnerability to sexual victimization: can reducing women's drinking prevent rape? *Substance Use and Misuse*, 44, 1349–1376.

University of Sterling, 2013. Health first: an evidence-based alcohol strategy for the UK. http://www.stir.ac.uk/media/schools/management/documents/Alcohol%20strategy.FINAL%20revision%202.pdf (accessed 14/05/2015).

Wagenaar, A.C., Tobler, A.L. and Komro, K.A., 2010. Effects of alcohol tax and price policies on morbidity and mortality: a systematic review. *American Journal of Public Health*, 100(11), 270–278.

Wagenaar, A.C., Livingstone, M.D. and Staras, S.S., 2015. Effects of a 2009 Illinois alcohol tax increase on fatal motor vehicle crashes. *American Journal of Public Health.* doi: 10.2105/AJPH.2014.302428.

White, H.R. and Jackson, K., 2004/2005. Social and psychological influences of emerging adult drinking behaviour. *Alcohol Research and Health*, 28(4), 182–190.

World Health Organization, 2009. *World Health Organization handbook for action to reduce alcohol-related harm.* http://www.euro.who.int/__data/assets/pdf_file/0012/43320/E92820.pdf (accessed 10/05/2014).

World Health Organization, 2014. *World Health Organization – global status report on alcohol and health.* http://www.who.int/substance_abuse/publications/global_alcohol_report/en/ (accessed 10/05/2015).

2 Alcohol and sport

Introduction

Despite the significant and wide-ranging harms associated with alcohol discussed in Chapter 1, according to Stainback (1997: 26):

> . . . alcohol, in particular beer, has played a significant role in sport. From the club rugby teams where beer drinking is an assumed after-game activity to an afternoon at the baseball park, consuming alcoholic beverages is a high profile activity in sport.

In this chapter, I argue that sport plays a significant and problematic role in normalizing alcohol use in general and excessive or binge drinking in particular. I will focus on three ways that sport plays its part. First, although there are certain restrictions on alcohol marketing, sport provides alcohol companies with a platform for promoting their brand and imprinting it on the sporting landscape and in the minds of potential customers, including children. Children watch sport and are bombarded with these brand images and logos. Research suggests that such marketing has a detrimental impact on the drinking habits of children and young people. Secondly, watching 'the game' is an occasion which licenses harmful drinking by fans and there is clear evidence that such game-related drinking (beyond the risks to the individual) contributes to disorder, aggression and violence, including domestic violence. Finally, I argue that sport encourages or normalizes the alcoholic binge among players. Excessive drinking is *the* choice for celebration, relaxation and team bonding in the sporting context.

Sponsorship

Despite the obvious incongruity between alcohol and sporting performance, sport has always played, and in many countries continues to play, a central role in brewers' marketing strategies. Sport provides access to millions of thirsty fans (customers) who traditionally consume beer (lager), particularly on 'game day'. According to Stainback (1997: 27), the success of the association between alcohol companies and sport is attributable to the fact that 'the demographics of beer drinkers and sports fans are largely synonymous'. According to Collins and

Vamplew (2002), the association between the drinks industry and sport stretches back to the birth of the latter in the UK during the nineteenth century. In particular, brewery families were instrumental in the formation of a number of cricket and rugby clubs. Liverpool FC owes its existence to the brewer John Houlding who founded the club in 1892, and with three other brewers controlled the club during its early years. Similarly, Manchester United FC owes its existence to a man called J.H. Davies, chairman of Manchester Breweries, who saved Newton Heath FC from liquidation in 1902, changed the club's name and provided £60 000 for a new ground at Old Trafford (Collins and Vamplew 2002). In the USA, the St Louis Cardinals were bought by August A. Busch, Jr., president of the Anheuser-Busch In Bev brewery, in 1953 (Stainback 1997). After the First World War, breweries in the UK were particularly keen to cultivate the well-being of their workforce and saw sport as an ideal vehicle. According to Stainback (1997: 42–43): 'Most breweries threw themselves and their money enthusiastically at the new vogue for providing sports facilities for their employees', which resulted in the formation of leagues and competitions between different companies (for example, London Breweries' Football League). This patronage was an early form of sponsorship.

Today, breweries and alcohol companies sponsor individuals, teams, competitions and even sporting stadiums by paying for the right to have their brand linked to, and displayed prominently, when a team/player performs.[1] The ultimate aim of brewers and distributors, of course, is to increase market share and revenue by getting more people to drink, and people who already drink to drink more or to switch brands. According to Hastings et al. (2010: 185): 'Sponsorship is a way of raising brand awareness, creating positive brand attitudes, and building emotional connections with consumers'. Furthermore Kelly et al. (2011:72) argue that 'image transfer' underpins sport sponsorship whereby the inherent positive (or admired) values of the activity (sport) are transferred to the sponsor. 'Specifically, image transfer in sport sponsorship mostly relates to values of being healthy, young, energetic, fast, vibrant and predominately masculine' (Kelly et al. 2011: 72). Collins and Vamplew (2002: 59) suggest that the model for modern sponsorship in the UK was established in the sport of darts in the 1930s, and by the late 1960s it was common to see sports events 'bearing the name of a drinks manufacturer or brand'. The sponsorship of teams (club and national) soon followed, for example, with Tennent's (lager) sponsorship of the Scottish national football team in the 1970s. Collins and Vamplew (2002) argue that in the UK in particular there was a significant class differentiation in terms of sponsorship. Wine and spirit manufacturers tended to focus on traditionally middle class sports whereas brewers targeted traditionally working class sports. For example, by sponsoring the glamorous sport of motor racing, Martini 'positioned itself as an aspirational drink for the affluent classes' (Collins and Vamplew 2002: 59), and champagne producers focused on sports such as polo and yachting.

Alcohol companies believe strongly that sport is a valuable marketing vehicle. According to O'Brien and Kypri (2008: 1961), '60% of all USA alcohol industry advertising dollars are spent on advertising during televised sports events'.

Perhaps a key aim of the association is to cultivate and promote brand identity, brand loyalty or generate brand capital which:

> . . . describes the accretion of meaning and emotion associated with a brand: this is one of the primary functions of marketing. The relationship which is established with a brand through marketing is ideally, from the marketer's point of view, a close one and brands are increasingly conceptualized as personalities with which we can form relationships. (Casswell 2004: 471)

Sport fans may develop a preference or loyalty for a particular brand or product because of its association with their sport, team or nation, and there is clear evidence that the association is profitable for both parties. In the USA, alcohol sponsorship features heavily in North American Association for Stock Car Auto Racing (NASCAR) racing, the National Football League (NFL), Major League Baseball (MLB) and the National Basketball Association (NBA), with the company Anheuser-Busch In Bev (which manufactures Budweiser and Bud Light) a prominent name. Between 1953 (the purchase of the Cardinals by Busch Jr.) and 1978, AB In Bev's brewery's annual sales grew by more than 500%, an increase partly attributed to the company's association with baseball (Stainback 1997). In the UK, alcohol has been closely associated with football, rugby, golf and cricket in various guises, with Guinness, Heineken, Carling and Carlsberg featuring prominently. Carlsberg is clear in terms of its goals:

> Beer and football go together – and we're doing all we can to make sure that the beer is Carlsberg! At every level of the game, Carlsberg has become the beer you associate with football . . . What's better than watching your favourite team with your best mates, while enjoying a cold pint of Carlsberg.[2]

In 2008, alcohol sponsorship of sport in the UK was worth over £300 million.[3] The Premier League (arguably the world's most commercially lucrative association football competition, established in 1993) was sponsored for over £1 million per month by Carling in 1998 (Collins and Vamplew 2002), and the parent company, Bass, reported that its sales of Carling lager increased by 31% to become UK's top selling alcohol brand (Carling sponsored the Premier League, or the Carling Premiership, between 1993 and 2001). Significant increases in sales were also reported by Carlsberg during its time as 'official beer' of the England football team. In Australia and New Zealand, rugby union, rugby league and cricket have all been sponsored by alcohol in various ways. Jones (2010) found that Australian alcohol companies spend $50 million a year on sport sponsorship. In addition to the high-profile sponsorship of elite sports alcohol companies, public houses, bars and local breweries sponsor amateur or student sport. For example, in the UK, Moet et Chandon 'hoped to establish drinking habits early through its sponsorship of public school cricket' (Collins and Vamplew 2002: 59), and in 1991 in the USA AB In Bev helped support more than 300 college teams and over 1000 other sporting events (Stainback 1997). In both these latter cases, those participating would not legally be allowed to buy the product of their sponsors (in most countries such practices are now forbidden). In Canada, however, Budweiser sponsor the Atlantic University League which means that in some states athletes under the legal drinking age of 19 years play for teams in that league.

Current situation

In the UK, the England football team have an 'official beer' supplier, Carlsberg, which also endorses development football competitions (the FA Carlsberg Vase, the FA Carlsberg Trophy and the FA Carlsberg Sunday Cup), and the Football Association's (FA's) premier cup competition was sponsored by Budweiser until 2014. Until recently, Carlsberg sponsored Liverpool FC and their rivals, Everton FC, are currently sponsored by Chang lager.[4] In Denmark, seven of the top ten premier league football clubs were sponsored by breweries in 2010, and in Germany all of the top ten premier league football clubs were sponsored by at least one German beer producer. The Union of European Football Association (UEFA) Champions League, Europe's premier club competition (the final in 2013 was the world's most watched annual sporting event that year), is prominently sponsored by Heineken. The World Cup, the most watched sporting event on earth, is sponsored by Budweiser. The England rugby union team have endorsement arrangements with Greene King Ale, which is the official beer of England rugby union and the official beer of Twickenham, the stadium where England play their home matches, and which sponsors the second division of club rugby in England. The premier rugby division was the Guinness Premiership until 2010. Wales, Scotland and Ireland rugby have associations with alcohol companies including Heineken, Guinness, S.A. Brain, Caledonia Best, Ginger Grouse and Bushmills Irish Whiskey, which serve as either 'official beer' or partners. Australian rugby union have Hahn Super Dry as their beer partner and St Hallett Barossa as their wine partner, and Victoria Bitter (VB) is the official beer of the National Rugby League and the shirt sponsor of the New South Wales Blues, and the Queensland Rugby League team is sponsored by XXXX ('four X'). The premier rugby union club competition in Europe was the Heineken Cup (an arrangement that ended in 2014). In cricket, the England and Wales Cricket Board (ECB) have Marston's Pedigree Bitter and Stowford Press English cider as partners and Veuve Clicquot as suppliers, and Castle Lager is a prominent sponsor of South Africa's cricket team. In the USA, AB In Bev was named Sports Sponsor of the Year in 2013, and their portfolio includes providing the official beer for the NFL, MLB, NBA, Professional Golfers' Association (PGA), Ladies Professional Golf Association (LPGA) and the Kentucky Derby. According to AB In Bev's website: 'Additional sponsorship include the No. 29 Budweiser Cheverolet SS, 95 local teams across four major sports leagues and dozens of running and cycling events nationwide'.[5] In 2011, the National Hockey League (NHL) secured sponsorship with MillerCoors in the USA and Molson Coors in Canada, worth $400 million over 7 years. The Executive Vice President of MillerCoors was clear about the rationale for the deal: 'Hockey fans are big beer drinkers. In fact we have data that shows hockey fans are the biggest beer drinkers of any major sports league'.[6] Formula One racing continues to allow alcohol brands to sponsor their sport, for example, Johnnie Walker, the whisky makers, sponsor McLaren, and Martini sponsor Williams, despite concerns about associating alcohol with driving.[7]

Jones (2010) argues that Lion Nathan, an Australian food company, created a new sport (or a new version of sport) purely to promote one of its alcohol brands. The XXXX Gold Beach Cricket Series (XXXX Gold being a brand of lager) was launched in 2006 and featured famous ex-players from Australia, England and the West Indies. According to Jones (2010), Lion Nathan spent 90% of XXXX Gold's marketing budget on the series and saw an increase in sales of 8% as a result. The particular ingenuity of the campaign meant that much of the money spent was clawed back through selling tickets, the television rights and other forms of merchandise. Andrew Coates, the director of the tournament, claimed that the tournament helped the product become the second best-selling beer in the country (Jones 2010).

The vast sums of money generated by sponsorship is an important funding stream for sport, not only at the elite level but at grass roots level too, helping to fund clubs, pay salaries, provide facilities and so forth. Some argue that the money from alcohol sponsorship is vital if sport is to flourish. Similar claims were voiced about tobacco sponsorship of sport. Tobacco funds have been replaced and perhaps alcohol sponsorship is also on the decline to be replaced in many cases by gambling companies.

An unhealthy alliance

In Chapter 1, we saw that the World Health Organization (WHO) was committed to a ban on alcohol advertising as a key part of harm reduction. In their European Charter on Alcohol, one of their key principles is that 'All children and adolescents have the right to grow up in an environment protected from the negative consequences of alcohol consumption and, to the extent possible, from the promotion of alcohol beverages' (WHO 2006: 23). In the UK, all television commercials for cigarettes were banned in 1965 with loose tobacco and cigar commercials following in 1991. It was not until 2003 that sponsorship of UK-based sporting events was banned, and in 2005 all tobacco branding was banned from appearing on UK television. The rationale behind the legislation was that any form of tobacco promotion encouraged smoking, and banning such promotion would be a significant harm-reduction intervention. There are growing calls for a similar stance to be taken in relation to alcohol. According to the Science Group of the European Alcohol and Health Forum (2009: 3), 'marketing communications are just one aspect of determinants of alcohol consumption and alcohol-related harm'. It is of course very difficult to isolate or prove that one variable (alcohol promotion) has a particular impact on alcohol consumption (and harm). Nevertheless, Saffer and Dave (2006) concluded that alcohol advertising bans decrease alcohol consumption, and Babor et al. (2010) report findings which suggest that awareness of, and liking of, alcohol advertisements, has an effect on intention to drink. Most studies exploring whether or not alcohol marketing influences alcohol consumption have focused on young people. The concern is that exposure to alcohol advertising will encourage young people to drink, or drink more. Austin et al. (2006: 382) found that children who are exposed to alcohol advertising progressively internalize messages that eventually impact behaviour. The first stage is that the advertisement is liked (funny, catchy, memorable), which is followed by a desire to emulate 'media portrayals of alcohol use' (identification), followed by coming to like beer brands and associate alcohol with positive experiences. According to Saffer and Dave (2006: 634), in relation to adolescents, 'alcohol advertising has a positive, but modest effect on annual alcohol participation, monthly participation and binge participation'. Smith and Foxcroft (2009: 9) conducted a systematic review of seven cohort studies on over 13 000 participants and found that 'exposure to alcohol advertising in young people influences their subsequent drinking behaviour', concluding that it 'is certainly plausible that advertising would have an effect on youth consumer behaviour . . .'. Hastings et al. (2010: 184) claim that advertising alcohol 'encourages young people to drink alcohol sooner and in greater quantities', and Ellickson et al. (2005: 235) found that several forms of alcohol advertising 'predict adolescent drinking'. Anderson et al. (2009: 242) found 'consistent evidence to link alcohol advertising with the uptake of drinking among non-drinking young people, and increased consumption among their drinking peers'. Waylen et al. (2015) found that exposure to alcohol use in films had an influence on drinking behaviour. They found that adolescents with the highest exposure to alcohol use in films were more likely to have tried alcohol, more likely to binge drink, more likely to drink weekly and more likely to have alcohol-related problems. Recent research in England and Scotland found that children as young as 10 years of age are familiar with alcohol brands, and boys in particular strongly associate football clubs and tournaments with beer brands such as Chang, Carlsberg and Carling that sponsor them.[8] Based on the available evidence about exposure to alcohol in the media, the Science Group of the European Alcohol and Health Forum (2009: 2) concluded that:

> Based on the consistency of findings across the studies, the confounders controlled for, the dose-response relationships, as well as the theoretical plausibility and experimental findings regarding the impact of media exposure and commercial communications, it can be concluded from the study reviews that alcohol marketing increases the likelihood that adolescents will start to use alcohol, and drink more if they are already using alcohol.

Given the concern about young people, coupled with the laws governing legal drinking age, there is a moral and legal duty for alcohol companies not to target youngsters through their marketing. Some countries, such as France, Russia and Norway, have gone further, seeking to protect all citizens from alcohol promotion by banning alcohol advertising altogether in almost all media. Sweden has strict limits on the types of alcohol product that can be advertised (only low-alcohol drinks). Singapore has legislated against alcohol advertising during children or family viewing times. Such restrictions are unpopular. According to Casswell

(1997: 251): 'Among those with a stake in alcohol industry profits, there is a reluctance to accept the use of public policies which have a direct impact on over-all consumption and drinking behaviour'. In the UK, such reluctance has resulted in a system of industry self-regulatory controls. The Portman Group, discussed in the previous chapter, has played its role in resisting potential profit-eroding legislation. The voluntary regulations put in place focus on the content of adver-tisements, the messages conveyed, timing and location of advertisements, and the media that can be used. The guiding principle in the UK is:

> Advertisements for alcoholic drinks should not be targeted at people under 18 years of age and should not imply, condone or encourage immoderate, irresponsible or anti-social drinking.[9]

The principle is fleshed out in terms of more than 20 rules and clauses giving further guidance about what is acceptable. For example, rule 18.3:

> Marketing communications must not imply that drinking alcohol is a key component of the success of a personal relationship or social event. The con-sumption of alcohol may be portrayed as sociable or thirst-quenching.[10]

And rule 18.4:

> Drinking alcohol must not be portrayed as a challenge. Marketing communi-cations must neither show, imply, encourage or refer to aggression or unruly, irresponsible or anti-social behaviour nor link alcohol with brave, tough or daring people or behaviour.[10]

These codes are fairly detailed and restrictive and can significantly hinder the marketing strategies and campaigns of alcohol companies. According to Casswell (2004: 472), restrictions are problematic for the industry because a key goal of alcohol marketing is:

> . . . to encourage and maintain new cohorts of drinkers in established alcohol markets. Natural attrition means a continual process of loss of heavy drinkers from the established market (through changes such as marriages and mort-gages, ageing and eventually death). The youth sector is an important part of the market as heavier drinking is concentrated in the late teenage years and in young adulthood.

Casswell (2004: 474) argues that voluntary codes can be ineffective. First, they only tend to cover the most visible of media (namely television) with the result that many producers are now targeting customers through social media platforms like Twitter and Facebook. Second, even if the codes are rigor-ously adhered to, they cannot counter 'the emotional impact of advertising'. In the UK, these codes now come under the Advertising Standards Authority

(ASA), another self-regulation organization.[11] There is evidence that both the spirit and the letter of the codes are often flouted. Tanski et al. (2015: 264) believe that 'marketing self-regulation has failed to keep television alcohol advertising from reaching large numbers of underage persons and affecting their drinking patterns'.

Sport sponsorship provides a loophole to circumvent some of the strict regulations, in particular the recommendations which specify that alcohol advertisements should not appear in broadcasts targeted at audiences below 18 years of age. Sport broadcasts (Super Bowl, World Cup, World Series and so on) are popular with children and young people and they make up a significant proportion of the audience. Consequently, they will be exposed to any marketing or advertising contained in broadcasts, at the stadiums and on any logos, hoardings and so forth. Moreover, they buy and wear team shirts which might display alcohol logos, and they collect posters, pictures and so on. Sponsors often interpret the letter of advertising/sponsorship regulation, even statutory laws, to their advantage. Even when faced with a ban on alcohol sponsorship, companies have managed to circumvent the spirit of the law. As mentioned, in France there is a complete ban on alcohol advertising, including sport sponsorship. This created a problem for teams which were sponsored by alcohol companies. The Welsh national rugby union team, who were sponsored by the brewer, S.A. Brain, were not allowed to display the Brains logo on their shirts while playing in France. Clever and inventive marketing executives thought up various alternatives to the logo, replacing it with 'Try Essai' in 2009, which was printed in the typeface and style of the original logo.[12] The Heineken Cup (a European rugby union competition) was referred to as the 'H Cup', with the 'H' appearing in the same livery as in the Heineken logo itself. According to Hastings et al. (2010: 186), there is a salutatory lesson to be learnt from the tobacco story. Before the outright ban, 'attempts to control content and adjust targeting simply resulted in more cryptic and imaginative campaigns', such as the Brains example above. They found evidence that the alcohol industry is explicitly engaged with strategies to circumvent the voluntary codes in order to both glamorize alcohol (make it 'cool') and target young people. Another strategy being used by alcohol companies to circumvent regulations is what is called 'brand stretching'. This is when alcohol brands produce a new category of product which carries the brand name, and any positive associations that has, with it. Carlsberg has been manufacturing and marketing an energy drink called Carlsberg Sport and has launched an initiative worth over 4 million Danish krone.[13]

The British Medical Association in the UK believes that the alcohol industry should be prohibited from sponsoring sport events and teams in order to limit the promotion of its products to young children and adults. It argues that:

> Sponsorship usually involves providing money to underwrite the event in return for having a logo prominently displayed or distributed on items such as caps and T-shirts and around the event venue. Children and adults become walking billboards when they wear these items.[14]

The Irish government recently dropped plans to ban the alcohol sponsorship of sport despite strong support for a change in the law. The minister who promoted the ban accused the government of putting business interest ahead of public health.[15]

The level of exposure to alcohol images, logos and references in sport can be significant. Graham and Adams (2013) conducted a frequency analysis of alcohol marketing and references to alcohol in televised English professional football during the 2011/2012 season. During that season three competitions had alcohol sponsors, namely the Budweiser FA Cup, the Carling League Cup and the UEFA Champions League sponsored by Heineken. They found that visual references to alcohol were common in the six matches they studied to the extent that there were 111.3 visual references per hour of broadcast (an average of nearly two a minute). Most were on hoardings advertising beer on and around the field of play, and a total of 17 alcohol commercials were broadcast during the games. Adams et al. (2014) studied broadcasts of the 2012 European Football Championships and found an average of 1.24 alcohol references per minute. Moreover, a recent study of the FIFA 2014 World Cup by Alcohol Concern found that viewers of an entire programme would be exposed to one alcohol reference per minute of playing time and around ten alcohol commercials for broadcasts by stations other than the non-commercial BBC. Alcohol Concern estimated that half of the games analysed would have been watched by over a million fans under 18 years.[16] Graham and Adams (2013: 5) conclude that current regulations 'make no attempt to restrict this constant bombardment or to make the case that association of alcohol with professional sport and sporting success is likely to reflect one aspect of social success'. In the USA, the Super Bowl is viewed by over 100 million people, which is great news for its sponsors and companies airing commercials during its broadcast. The commercials have become an event in themselves with many saying the commercials are their main reason for watching.[17] The audience contains millions of children and some believe that alcohol companies target young people in the design of their commercials.[18] The use of social media to supplement television and other advertising of alcohol is also seen as a particular risk to young people and children in the formation of drinking habits and cultures.[19]

Grass roots

It is not only at the elite professional level that alcohol companies sponsor sport. Alcohol also has a negative and often more clearly demonstrable impact at grass roots level. Amateur clubs are often sponsored by a local public house or local brewery that provides the athletes with a supply of free or discounted alcohol. O'Brien and Kypri (2008: 1961) found that in New Zealand:

> Alcohol industry sponsorship of sportspeople, and in particular the provision of free or discounted alcoholic beverages, is associated with hazardous drinking after adjustment for a range of potential confounders.

Research by O'Brien (2014) found that 36% of UK university sportspeople received some form of alcohol sponsorship (such as money, travel costs, free drinks or use of venue) from alcohol-related companies (such as public houses and shops). Those in receipt of such sponsorship were likely to drink more alcohol and were at a higher risk of hazardous drinking. O'Brien (2014: 2) concludes that: 'Alcohol industry sponsorship is associated with more problematic drinking in UK university sportspeople'. There are other concerns related to alcohol promotion in the context of sport. Marketing campaigns often target a particular constituency (young men) and, in doing so, sexualized images are often used, which reinforce a particular brand of masculine identity while objectifying and sexualizing women. According to Weaving (2009), Coors Light and Budweiser are particularly guilty of this type of marketing strategy in Canada.

Power and influence

Not only are alcohol companies able to manipulate sport for marketing purposes, it seems that they are able, through their commercial activities and influence on sports governing bodies, to change the laws of countries in their favour. The Fédération Internationale de Football Association (FIFA), which organizes the World Cup, have a record of promoting the interests of its commercial partners, which include Budweiser, 'the official beer'. AB InBev, owner of Budweiser, pays 'anything between $10 and $25 million a year to be part of the World Cup "family"' (Gornall 2014: 16). Brazil, the country hosting the World Cup in 2014, was obliged by FIFA to waive the taxes on any profits made by sponsors during the World Cup. Gornall argues that in 2014 this obscene condition left 'sponsors such as Budweiser free to walk away with every *Real* they pocket[ed], depriving Brazil of an estimated £312 million in revenue' (Gornall 2014: 15). The poorer people of Brazil bore the cost of those tax breaks. Planned increases on alcohol tax were also postponed until after the tournament and Brazilian laws banning alcohol from sports stadiums were abandoned. Gornall (2014: 16) quotes Ronaldo Laranjeira, Professor of Psychiatry at the University of São Paulo, who said that it was shocking that FIFA:

> . . . can come to a country and makes [sic] it change its laws. We have been very active in trying to embarrass the government on this issue, but in the end the alcohol industry has won. At the moment it is running the show . . . .

Budweiser will be the sponsors of the World Cup in both 2018 and 2022, in Russia and Qatar respectively. The Winter Olympic Games at Sochi were alcohol-free (part of the Russian government's efforts to curb a national alcohol problem) and Qatar is a strict Muslim country with tight alcohol regulations. Gornall (2014) observes that Qatar has already agreed to sell alcohol in 'fan zones' in 2022 and wonders whether Russia will change its approach in the face of FIFA pressure in 2022.[20]

Alcohol and watching sport

Many of the products marketed through sport are actually consumed by sports fans when watching sport, either live or on television. According to Johnson (1988), beer and sport are inseparable in the American lexicon. Collins and Vamplew (2002: 69) argue that: 'It is no exaggeration to suggest that, no matter what the sport or its level of popularity, the consumption of alcohol is almost an intrinsic part of the spectator experience'. Kahn (2007: 3) argues that beer and baseball are particularly closely connected in many ways, including sponsorship and consumption by players, but especially in terms of its consumption by fans at games: 'There isn't a more clear connection between beer and baseball than the sight of overflowing cups of beer being passed by fans – including children – down rows of seats'. Furthermore, he claims that the relationship between alcohol and American sport undermines public health efforts to educate citizens about the problems relating to alcohol. No wonder then that alcohol companies spend billions of dollars targeting this population. In the UK, in the latter part of the nineteenth century, the temperance movement was particularly hostile towards sport because of its close association with alcohol and the associated licentiousness and immorality (Collins and Vamplew 2002). The close association continues to this day and there are a number of problems associated with fan culture for which alcohol is a key contributory factor. Drinking a lot of alcohol on match day is a long-standing and continuing tradition among a constituency of fans before, during and after matches, and heavy drinking among fans often results in problems.

In the late twentieth century, and perhaps less visibly in the early twenty-first century, there has been high-profile concern about the behaviour of some fans (hooligans), particularly, but by no means exclusively, in relation to association football in the UK and Europe. Infamous examples (and there are plenty more) include rioting at Heysel Stadium in Belgium in 1985, and trouble at the FIFA World Cup in France in 1998. Lenk et al. (2009: 451) argue that in the USA there have been a number of 'high-profile alcohol-related violent incidents at professional sports stadiums in recent years'. An example of disorder in the USA is the violence and vandalism by fans following the San Francisco Giants World Series victory over the Detroit Tigers in 2012. It has been alleged that alcohol and its availability has played a crucial causal role in this kind of sport-related disorder. Dunning et al. (1988) and others have questioned whether the phenomenon of spectator disorder, violence or rioting can be attributed simply to the consumption of alcohol. Clearly alcohol cannot be the only cause of spectator violence, but it undeniably increases risks. In the UK, alcohol, or access to it, by fans, particularly football fans, remains an issue for governing bodies and the police alike. In 1985, the Sporting Events Act (Control of Alcohol etc.) came into force in the UK. Among other things, the act prohibits the consumption of alcohol within view of the playing area from 15 minutes before the event starts, to 15 minutes after it finishes. Other laws prohibit the consumption of alcohol on buses and trains carrying fans to matches, and certain games between bitter rivals with a track record of disorder might be scheduled earlier in the day so as to minimize the 'drinking time' available to fans before the game starts. UEFA does not allow the sale of alcohol at stadiums during its competitions (executive sections are exempt), which led to the paradoxical situation 'where Heineken beer sponsors the UEFA Champions League tournament under the slogan, "Heineken and the Champions League: Great Together", but at which their product is not permitted to be consumed by non-executive supporters' (Pearson and Sale 2011: 155).

The merit of such legislation, and the evidence on which it is based, is disputed. 'Indeed, when one looks at other sport, the alleged causal link between heavy drinking and violence is untenable' (Collins and Vamplew 2002: 86). Yet, as mentioned in the opening chapter, there is significant evidence which suggests that being drunk increases the likelihood that one might commit, or become a victim of, violent crime, and it would be strange if football fans were immune to these problems. The Institute of Alcohol Studies reports that alcohol is present in over half of all crime committed in the UK and that a high proportion of victims of violent crime have been drinking at the time of the incident. In the year April 2004 to March 2005 37% of offenders had a problem with alcohol use and the figures were the same for binge drinking. Moreover, alcohol was found to be a factor in 75% of stabbings, 70% of beatings and 50% of fights and domestic assaults.[21] In the USA, over a 4 year period, 38% of individuals involved in violent incidents were under the influence of alcohol at the time (Giesbrecht et al. 2010). Given that these are the types of crime associated with fan disorder, it would be disingenuous to exclude alcohol from the mix of antecedent causes. Thirty three per cent of all football-related arrests in the UK during the 2010/2011 season were for alcohol-related offences.[22] Lenk et al. (2009) presented data on the frequency and type of complaints received by law enforcement agencies in relation to sport stadiums in the USA. The most common types of complaint were about fights inside and outside the stadiums and problems with intoxicated fans.

Although the causal role of alcohol in sport-related disorder is disputed, meta-analysis research by Bushman and Cooper (1990) found that alcohol does cause aggressive behaviour. Matthews et al. (2006: 667) found that 'major sports events, which engage the national population, produce a significant increase in assault related injury' and this is partly attributable to alcohol consumption among spectators. Moore et al. (2007: 119) argue that: 'Alcohol, aggression and assault injury are strongly associated with popular sporting events'. The consumption of alcohol by spectators, coupled with other aspects of watching sport (animosity between opposing fans, being in a large crowd, opportunities for confrontation), can lead to aggression and violence among spectators. Sivarajasingham et al. (2005) found that in relation to international soccer and rugby matches, assault injury resulting in hospital treatment was higher when the home team won than when they lost. Moore et al. (2007) found that post-match alcohol consumption, which leads to violence and disorder, is driven by aggression. They also found that their team winning was more likely to increase fan aggression which in turn fuelled drinking, 'an observation which is consistent with psychological models of aggression' (Moore et al. 2007: 124). Many sports have tried to cultivate a more family-friendly ethos at stadiums, but such an ethos is always fragile when fans are drunk or drinking.

The association of sport and alcohol is by no means restricted to watching professional sport. Glassman et al. (2010: 417) found that in the USA students are particularly prone to problematic drinking on 'game day'. Their results showed that 'nearly 2 out of every 5 students engaged in heavy episodic drinking on game day', which puts them at significant risk of a number of negative alcohol-related consequences, including driving under the influence, getting injured, being involved in violence, being victimized sexually and getting into trouble with the police. In the UK in 2013 British Universities and Colleges Sport (BUCS) implemented a policy to try and tackle some of the alcohol-related problems associated with watching and playing sport at university. Increasing incidences of drunken spectators and anti-social behaviour of fans led to the creation of a code of conduct which included the 'right to refuse entry or exclude any supporters arriving or in attendance at BUCS events under the influence of alcohol or demonstrating anti-social behaviour'.[23]

Another problem associated with excessive alcohol consumption while watching sport is domestic violence. The Institute of Alcohol Studies found that alcohol had been consumed prior to the offence in nearly three quarters (73%) of domestic violence cases and was a feature in 62% in the UK.[24] In England there has been a recognized pattern of increased levels of domestic violence surrounding major football tournaments which involve the national team. Watching important football matches on television is associated with higher levels of alcohol consumption. Sales of alcohol in the UK during the 2014 World Cup totalled £1.1 billion, £15.1 million more than the same period in 2013.[25] Moreover, police records show that when England beat Slovenia, and when they lost to Germany in the 2010 World Cup, reports of domestic violence increased by 27% and 29% respectively.[26] The matter is of course more complex than watching sport or the quantity of alcohol consumed; nevertheless, it illustrates some of the less obvious consequences (for some) of excessive drinking.

Celebrating with alcohol

The final idea I want to explore in this chapter is the role sport plays in normalizing excessive drinking as celebration. In many cultures, alcohol is the cornerstone of celebration and one could argue that sport simply mirrors this. However, given the need to reduce 'risky' alcohol consumption I believe that the use of alcohol in sporting celebrations is problematic. Athletes are supposed to be fit, healthy and strong, both mentally and physically. It often comes as a surprise to hear that they engage in unhealthy behaviours such as smoking, drinking and taking drugs, yet such behaviour is more common than we think. Contemporary elite sport is, as has been widely documented, a global commercial phenomenon where the profit motive and athletic excellence are arguably equally important. There is pressure to succeed and the price of failure can, and is often measured in, millions of dollars or pounds. Recent advances in sport science and the increasingly commercial nature of modern sport has seen significant changes in athletic lifestyles and attitudes towards alcohol consumption, particularly in relation to its impact on performance.[27] According to Collins and Vamplew (2002) there was a time when alcohol was an important part of an athlete's routine; for example, it was thought to provide extra courage for boxers in the nineteenth century. Its use was not limited to boxing, however. 'In his *Principles of Training for Amateur Athletics* of 1892 H.L. Curtis suggested moderate consumption of alcohol as part of a sportsman's regime, but warned against smoking and coffee' (Collins and Vamplew 2002: 92). According to Collins and Vamplew (2002), the American College of Sports Medicine's research in 1982, highlighted the negative physiological and psychomotor consequences of its consumption for athletes, and subsequent studies have led to most elite athletes eschewing alcohol, particularly during important training and competition periods. Moreover, most professional (and amateur) teams will be expected to moderate or eliminate their alcohol consumption at certain occasions.

One obvious exemption is in celebration. It continues to be part of the sporting ritual to present winners with a magnum of champagne, the contents of which are usually sprayed over teammates, coaches and fans, rather than consumed. Successful Formula One racing drivers drench each other on the podium following a Grand Prix. Football, hockey, rugby and cricket teams soak each other with bottles of champagne in an almost scripted celebratory routine, jumping up and down, singing and, of course, obligatorily drinking of alcohol from the trophy itself.[28] Sponsors often provide a ready supply of beer for players to drink on the pitch, and awards for man of the match (most valuable player) consist of a bottle of champagne. Of course, it is not just sporting achievements where alcohol is present; in certain cultures it is *de rigueur* to accompany most celebrations with some form of alcohol. It seems inconceivable that one can celebrate anything without a drink. In May 2013, Wigan Athletic FC (rank outsiders at the beginning of the tournament) won the prestigious FA Cup in England, an occasion which usually demands the consumption of alcohol. Given they had to play another crucial game a few days later they had to curb any celebrations. Pundits and commentators seemed perplexed about how they would celebrate without alcohol. Members of Arsenal FC's 2015 FA Cup winning side were out celebrating until 6 am following their victory. A few hours later they took the traditional open-top bus ride through the streets of North London to show celebrate with the fans and show off the trophy. During the parade Jack Wilshere, a player with a history of disciplinary problems, was drinking alcohol and sang offensive songs about Tottenham Hotspur FC, Arsenal's bitter rivals[29] (he was subsequently fined £40 000 by the FA for bringing the game into disrepute and severely warned about his future conduct).[30]

The year 2012 was particularly successful in terms of British sport, perhaps the most successful ever. There are two particular examples of success which perhaps illustrate the close association between success and alcohol. The first is Bradley Wiggins, who became the first Briton to win what some argue is the ultimate sporting contest, the Tour de France. He subsequently won a gold medal at the London Olympic Games. The second example is Andy Murray, the British tennis player who arguably reached similar heights by winning a Grand Slam championship for the first time (the US Open) having won the Olympic singles gold medal a short time previously. They are obviously very different types of sport, and Wiggins and Murray are very different characters who cultivate (or at least have) very different public images. It was interesting to observe how the discourse around both these incredible successes played out in the British media in terms of relationships with alcohol.

Bradley Wiggins is a popular figure and is different to other elite endurance athletes in many ways. He seems to cultivate an image and persona akin to British indie rock icons like Paul Weller and Liam Gallagher. His chosen profession of course necessitates a very different lifestyle to a rock star, involving disciplined training, a carefully controlled diet and often long periods of abstinence from alcohol. Given the demands of cycling, diet and weight are crucial for success, and abstaining from calorific alcohol for a long period of time is common. It is perhaps expected that a period of abstinence will be broken by a 'blow out' and many athletes report bingeing, not only on alcohol but also on food once the competition is over. Wiggins celebrated his gold medal at the Olympic Games by drinking vodka and tonic (perhaps to reduce the calorie intake). Andrew Brown, writing in *The Times* after Wiggins' gold medal victory in the Olympic time trial opined that:

> We shouldn't be surprised that Bradley Wiggins 'tied one on' [a colloquialism for getting drunk] last night after winning the gold medal in the time trial yesterday. He competes in a sport that involves lengthy periods of strict self-denial and exceedingly rigorous training, so after all that is finished there's understandably an urge to let the hair down, release tension- and drink thirstily . . . . They nearly always abstain from alcohol during training. When the contest is over, however, these sportsmen permit themselves a full-blown fiesta – rather like the feasts that punctuate the religious calendar.[31]

Alcohol featured many times in the discourse surrounding Wiggins' success. As a topic, it played an important role in connecting with the fans and galvanizing his image as 'a down-to-earth working class lad'. He joked with the crowd on the winner's podium at the Tour de France, warning them, 'don't get too drunk'.[32] In December 2012, Wiggins was voted BBC Sports Personality of the Year (a very prestigious award decided by public vote). Alcohol was at the forefront of his involvement in the event. In his acceptance speech he made reference to the 'free bar' after the show, he later joined a band on stage at the after show party, drink in hand and invited people to 'have a drink on him', adding 'I've got my credit card behind the bar if anyone wants a drink'.[33] Later on in the evening/early next morning he was photographed leaving a nightclub bleary eyed, and then again at a fast food restaurant at 5 am, which seemed to give him further 'street cred' among fans and the media. A dominant attitude towards Wiggins was that such a celebration, involving excessive consumption of alcohol, was not only acceptable, but deserved and laudable. The coverage was almost wholly positive and uncritical of the behaviour, despite the persecution of similar behaviour among other constituents by the media, for example, students, young women and certain celebrities. His status as a champion and hero seemed to immunize him from media scorn. Given the magnitude of his achievements in 2012 it might seem churlish to problematize the purportedly harmless and deserved celebration, but Wiggins himself recently revealed in his autobiography that there was a period in his life, early in his career, where alcohol was a problem. Simon Hattenstone, writing in the UK's *Guardian* broadsheet newspaper, talked to Wiggins about these issues:

> 'I probably get my addictive streak from my father', he has said previously. Before long he'd be at his local for opening time every day. Often he'd get through 12 pints in a day. 'I was just bored shitless and didn't know what to do.' He says many athletes experience depression after great victories – it's the anti-climax. The bender lasted nine months.[34]

I will pick up on these issues later in the book, but it is interesting to contrast Wiggins with another 2012 British sporting hero. At the 2012 US Open tennis tournament the British player Andy Murray won his first major title, and the UK's first in men's tennis for 76 years. The achievement was, quite rightly, a cause for celebration for Murray and his family, friends and supporters. It was notable (at least to me) that the media focused on Murray's abstinence from alcohol, and there was general incredulity that he was not going to imbibe at this most significant of career moments. It was widely reported that Murray refused his friends' and family's attempts to get him to drink. The UK's *Telegraph* broadsheet newspaper reported that the tab for Murray's celebration party at a New York restaurant ran to $6500, of which Murray's contribution amounted to one soft drink costing $6.[35]

As has been mentioned, attitudes towards the celebrations of athletes are not always so generous. At the 2010 Winter Olympic Games in Vancouver, the alcohol-fuelled celebrations of the Canadian women's ice hockey team came in for some criticism. Edwards et al. (2013) argue that gender double standards were at play which seemed to condone, if not encourage, the use of alcohol by male athletes in sport to celebrate important victories, but which condemned the same or similar behaviour in women. Edwards et al. (2013) illustrate the double standards by citing the example of Jon Montgomery, a Canadian gold medallist who was filmed accepting and drinking a pitcher of beer from spectators live on television.

Significantly, Montgomery received no criticism for his actions from the media or even from the International Olympic Committee (IOC). Stories of male athletes engaging in similar post-game activities abound, but such incidents are rarely criticized or admonished. Celebrating victory with excessive drinking is simply customary in male sporting practices. In fact, such behaviour is usually celebrated as a 'time-honoured tradition' within the sporting community (Edwards et al. 2013: 688).

Of course, drinking underage, drinking before important matches and athletes with a track record of alcohol misuse may all experience levels of scrutiny by the media, but the practice of celebrating victories with alcohol remains a central plank of sporting narratives. The autobiographies of various athletes include, or at least allude to, accounts of celebrating with as much enthusiasm as the victory itself. In fact, the salacious stories of what went on out of sight are part of the appeal of such books. Coverage of the recent 2014 Ryder Cup victory by Europe had its fair share of questions about 'how long did the party last?', 'how was the head?' and other references to alcohol. I will return to some of the issues raised in this last section in the next chapter where I say more about the alcohol ethos of sport and its consequences. It suffices for now to claim that watching sport cultivates and/or galvanizes the idea that celebration *must* involve the use, and preferably the excessive use, of alcohol. Winning at sport means that you deserve to get drunk.

Summary

In this chapter, I have argued that the relationship between sport and alcohol is morally problematic because of the role sport plays in the promotion and normalization of its use. I have focused on the way in which alcohol companies use sport to market and promote their product, which is particularly problematic with respect to exposing young people and children to alcohol imagery and branding. I have also described some of the problems that arise among fans when they watch sport either in the stadium or at home. Finally, I argued that the message from sport is that getting drunk and binge drinking are legitimate and deserved after winning in sport (or indeed for drowning one's sorrows after a loss). In the next chapter I will explore the alcohol ethos in sport in more detail.

Notes

1 In the UK, the home of Surrey County Cricket Club and the England test match venue 'The Oval,' was branded 'the Fosters Oval' from 1989 to 2000; in Ontario, Canada, the London Nights Hockey team play at 'Budweiser Gardens', and for a period of time, the English non-league football club Witton Albion's ground was called the 'Bargain Booze Stadium'.
2 Taken from page 1 of 'Alcohol and football', a briefing by Alcohol Concern. http://www.alcoholconcern.org.uk/wp-content/uploads/woocommerce_uploads/2014/10/Alcohol-and-Football_Briefing.pdf (accessed 12/05/2015).
3 http://www.publications.parliament.uk/pa/cm201213/cmselect/cmhealth/132/132vw20.htm#footnote_2 (accessed 11/04/2013).
4 In the UK, the state-owned television channel, the BBC has, since its inception, been commercial-free. Through sponsoring sport, companies, including alcohol companies (and until 2005, tobacco companies), could market and promote their product on the BBC. For over 30 years the World Snooker Championship, televised by the BBC, was the Embassy (cigarette) World Championship.
5 http://anheuser-busch.com/index.php/anheuser-busch-named-sports-business-journal-2013-sports-sponsor-of-the-year/ (accessed 3/10/2014).
6 http://www.nytimes.com/2011/02/23/sports/hockey/23beer.html?_r=1& (accessed 3/10/2014).
7 http://www.telegraph.co.uk/sport/motorsport/formulaone/11226082/FIA-president-Jean-Todt-under-fire-for-failure-to-ban-alcohol-sponsorship-in-Formula-One.html (accessed 5/05/2015).

8 http://www.alcoholconcern.org.uk/wp-content/uploads/woocommerce_
   uploads/2015/02/Childrens-Recognition-of-Alcohol-Marketing_Briefing.compressed.
   pdf (accessed 1/05/2015).
9 http://www.cap.org.uk/advertising-codes/broadcast/codeitem?cscid={dafa8794-505f-
   4d15-ba5d-d0b8cf1507e7}#.VVHTBPlVhBd (accessed 12/05/2015).
10 http://www.asa.org.uk/News-resources/Hot-Topics/Alcohol.aspx (accessed
   3/10/2014).
11 Alcohol Concern found posters advertising alcohol on many bus stops outside schools
   in Cardiff, UK, despite pledges by the alcohol industry not to advertise in such locations.
   http://www.alcoholconcern.org.uk/projects/alcohol-concern-cymru/news/worries-
   over-alcohol-adverts-outside-cardiff-schools (accessed 16/10/2014).
12 Scoring a 'try' is worth 5 pints in rugby union and is the goal of the game (equivalent to
   touch down). The French word is *essai*. S.A. Brain produces a brand of ale called S.A.,
   so the shirt logo 'Try Essai' was an invitation to 'Try S.A.'.
13 http://news.cision.com/dk/mark---lindberg-a-s/r/sponsormillioner-fra-carlsberg-sport-
   til-den-lokale-idraet,c9131200 (accessed 16/10/2014).
14 http://bma.org.uk/news-views-analysis/news/2012/july/bma-calls-for-alcohol-spon-
   sorship-ban (accessed 11/04/2010).
15 http://www.irishtimes.com/news/politics/alcohol-sponsorship-bill-dropped-1.2077768
   (accessed 2/05/2015).
16 http://www.alcoholconcern.org.uk/wp-content/uploads/woocommerce_
   uploads/2014/10/Alcohol-Marketing-at-the-FIFA-World-Cup-2014_pdf.pdf (accessed
   12/09/2015).
17 http://www.mediapost.com/publications/article/242856/half-of-americans-watch-
   super-bowl-for-the-ads.html?edition=79820 (accessed 1/05/2015).
18 http://www.iogt.org/eastasiaupdate/84/nfl-super-bowl-a-lot-is-on-the-line-tonight/
   (accessed 1/05/2015).
19 http://alcoholresearchuk.org/news/constructing-alcohol-identities-the-role-of-social-
   network-sites-sns-in-young-peoples-drinking-cultures/ (accessed 1/05/2015).
20 In 2012, the then chairman of the English Premier League, Sir Dave Richards, reacted
   badly to FIFA awarding the 2022 World Cup to Qatar and the accompanying threat of
   an alcohol-free tournament. Much to the embarrassment of his employers, he ranted
   that drinking 'is our culture as much as your culture is not drinking'. He subsequently
   stumbled into the hotel fountain, allegedly under the influence of alcohol. http://
   www.theguardian.com/football/2012/mar/14/dave-richards-fifa-uefa-stole-football
   (accessed 23/10/2014).
21 http://www.ias.org.uk/resources/factsheets/crime.pdf (accessed 15/04/20013).
22 http://socialwelfare.bl.uk/subject-areas/services-activity/criminal-justice/
   homeoffice/141854fbo_season_2011_121.pdf (accessed 15/04/2013).
23 http://www.uwesu.org/pageassets/sports/BUCS_anti-social_behaviour_and_
   initiations_policy_-_October_2013.pdf (accessed 20/11/2013).
24 http://www.community-safety.info/24.html (accessed 23/10/2014).
25 http://www.talkingretail.com/category-news/industry-announcements/report-shows-
   beer-main-winner-world-cup-campaign/ (accessed 5/05/2015).
26 Cafe, R., 2012. Euro 2012: tournament football and domestic violence. http://www.
   bbc.co.uk/news/ukengland-18379093 (accessed 21/12/2012).
27 Research by Prentice et al. (2014) showed only limited performance reductions after 'a
   heavy night on the beer'.
28 The USA soccer team participated in such a celebration on hearing they had qualified
   for the 2014 World Cup. http://www.huffingtonpost.com/2013/09/11/us-soccer-omar-
   gonzalez-chugs-beer_n_3904225.html (accessed 23/10/2014).
29 http://www.dailymail.co.uk/sport/football/article-3104529/Jack-Wilshere-leads-
   celebrations-Arsenal-stars-party-night-second-consecutive-FA-Cup-victory-Wembley.
   html (accessed 9/07/2015).

30 http://www.bbc.co.uk/sport/0/football/33171493 (accessed 8/07/2015).
31 Brown, A., 2012. Bradley Wiggins: no wonder he decided to celebrate with vodka-and-tonics. *The Telegraph*, 2 August. http://blogs.telegraph.co.uk/news/andrewmcfbrown/100174091/bradley-wiggins-no-wonder-he-decided-to-celebrate-with-vodka-and-tonics/ (accessed 19/12/2012).
32 http://www.cyclingweekly.co.uk/news/latest-news/bradley-wiggins-quotes-our-pick-of-the-best-166580 (accessed 12/05/2015).
33 http://www.bbc.co.uk/sport/0/sports-personality/20767828 (accessed 2/04/2013).
34 http://www.guardian.co.uk/sport/2012/nov/02/bradley-wiggins-interview-tour (accessed 20/11/2012).
35 Hughes, M., 2012. Andy Murray: victory is payback for family's sacrifices. *The Telegraph*, 12 September. http://www.telegraph.co.uk/sport/tennis/andymurray/9538075/Andy-Murray-Victory-is-payback-for-familys-sacrifices.html (accessed 12/12/2012).

References

Adams, J., Coleman, J. and White, M., 2014. Alcohol marketing in televised international football: frequency analysis. *BMC Public Health*, 14: 473.

Anderson, P., et al., 2009. Impact of alcohol advertising and media exposure on adolescent alcohol use: a systematic review of longitudinal studies. *Alcohol and Alcoholism*, 44(3), 229–243.

Austin, E.W., Chen, M.-J. and Grube, J.W., 2006. How does alcohol advertising influence underage drinking? The role of desirability, identification and scepticism. *Journal of Adolescent Health*, 38, 376–384.

Babor, T., et al., 2010. *Alcohol: no ordinary commodity—research and public policy*, 2nd edn. Oxford: Oxford University Press.

Bushman, B.J. and Cooper, H.M., 1990. Effects of alcohol on human aggression: and integrative research review. *Psychological Bulletin*, 107(3), 341–354.

Casswell, S., 1997. Public discourse on alcohol. *Health Promotion International*, 12(3), 251–257.

Casswell, S., 2004. Alcohol brands in young people's everyday lives: new developments in marketing, *Alcohol and Alcoholism*, 39(6), 471–476.

Collins, T. and Vamplew, W., 2002. *Mud, sweat and beers: a cultural history of sport and alcohol*. Oxford: Berg.

Dunning, E., Murphy, P. and Williams, J.M., 1988. *The roots of football hooliganism*. London: Routledge & Keegan Paul.

Edwards, L., Jones, C. and Weaving, C., 2013. Celebration on ice: double standards following the Canadian women's gold medal victory at the 2010 Winter Olympics. *Sport in Society*, 16(5), 682–698.

Ellickson, P., et al., 2005. Does alcohol advertising promote adolescent drinking? Results from a longitudinal study. *Addiction*, 100, 235–246.

Giesbrecht, N., Cukier, S. and Steeves, D., 2010. Collateral damage from alcohol: implications of 'second –hand effects of drinking' for populations and health priorities. *Addiction*, 105(8), 1323–1325.

Glassman, T.J., et al., 2010. Extreme ritualistic alcohol consumption among college students on game day. *Journal of American College Health*, 58(5), 413–423.

Gornall, J., 2014. World Cup 2014: festival of football or alcohol? *British Medical Journal*, 348, 15–17.

Graham, A. and Adams, J., 2013. Alcohol marketing in televised English professional football: a frequency analysis. *Alcohol and Alcoholism*, 1–6. doi: 10.1093/alcalc/agt140.

Hastings, G., et al., 2010. Alcohol advertising: the last chance saloon, *British Medical Journal*, 340, 184–186.

Johnson, W.O., 1988. Sports and suds: the beer business and the sports world have brewed up a potent partnership. *Sports Illustrated*, 69, 68–82.

Jones, S.C., 2010. When does alcohol sponsorship of sport become sports sponsorship of alcohol? A case study of developments in sports in Australia. *International Journal of Sports Marketing and Sponsorship*, 11(3), 250–261.

Kahn, J.P., 2007. Baseball, alcohol and public health. *American Journal of Bioethics*, 7(7), 3.

Kelly, P., et al., 2011. Charismatic cops, patriarchs and a few good women: leadership, club culture and young peoples' drinking. *Sport, Education and Society*, 16(4), 467–484.

Lenk, K.M., Toomey, T.L. and Erickson, D.J., 2009. Alcohol-related problems and enforcement at professional sports stadiums. *Drugs: Education, Prevention and Policy*, 16(5), 451–462.

Matthews, K., Shepherd, J. and Sivarajasingham, V., 2006. Violence related injury and the price of beer in England and Wales. *Applied Economics*, 38, 661–670.

Moore, S.C., et al., 2007. The effect of rugby match outcome on spectator aggression and intention to drink alcohol. *Criminal Behaviour and Mental Health*, 17, 118–127.

O'Brien, K.S., 2014. Alcohol industry sponsorship and hazardous drinking in UK university sport. Final report for Alcohol Research UK. http://alcoholresearchuk.org/downloads/finalReports/FinalReport_0112.pdf (accessed 10/02/2015).

O'Brien, K.S. and Kypri, K., 2008. Alcohol sponsorship and hazardous drinking among sportspeople. *Addiction*, 103, 1961–1966.

Pearson, G. and Sale, A., 2011. On the lash – revisiting the effectiveness of alcohol controls at football matches. *Policing and Society*, 21(2), 150–166.

Saffer, H. and Dave, D., 2006. Alcohol advertising and alcohol consumption by adolescents. *Health Economics*, 15, 617–637.

Science Group of the European Alcohol and Health Forum, 2009. Does marketing communication impact on the volume and patterns of consumption of alcoholic beverages, especially by young people? A review of longitudinal studies. http://ec.europa.eu/health/ph_determinants/life_style/alcohol/Forum/docs/science_o01_en.pdf (accessed 12/03/02015).

Sivarajasingham, V., Moore, S. and Shepherd, J.P., 2005. Winning, losing and violence. *Injury Prevention*, 11, 69–70.

Smith, L.A. and Foxcroft, D.R., 2009. The effect of alcohol advertising, marketing and portrayal on drinking behaviour in young people: systematic review of prospective cohort studies. *BMC Public Health*, 9, 51. doi: 10.1186/1471-2458-9-51.

Stainback, R.D., 1997. *Alcohol and sport*. Champaign, IL: Human Kinetics.

Tanski, S.E., et al., 2015. Cued recall of alcohol advertising on television and underage drinking. *JAMA Pediatrics*, 169(3), 264–271.

Waylen, A., et al., 2015. Alcohol use in films and adolescent alcohol use. *JAMA Pediatrics*, 135(5), doi: 10.1542/peds.2014–2978.

Weaving, C., 2009. Are you man enough for the Mystery Mansion?: An analysis of the connections between leisure experiences, sex and beer company promotions. Paper presented to the 37th International Association for the Philosophy of Sport Conference. Seattle University, Seattle, Washington, 27–30 August.

World Health Organization, 2006. Framework for alcohol policy in the WHO European region. http://www.euro.who.int/__data/assets/pdf_file/0007/79396/E88335.pdf (accessed 10/02/2015).

3 Sport and its alcohol ethos

Introduction

Alcohol was used in the past, and in some cases might still be used, as a form of performance enhancement, for example to calm nerves, provide courage and so on. These days it is largely accepted that alcohol is detrimental to sporting performance. Consequently, in the overwhelming majority of cases alcohol consumption in sport is now a social rather than a sporting issue (Collins and Vamplew 2002). In this chapter I argue that alcohol continues to play a central role in modern sport, even at the elite professional level. Despite its deleterious effects on performance, health and reputation, its consumption remains a core part of the sporting ethos. Sportsmen and women at all levels drink to celebrate, to relax, to bond with teammates and to relieve stress. Unfortunately, many drink excessively on occasion and come to the public's attention through the media, which seems to have a veracious appetite for alcohol-related scandal. Individuals who get into trouble through alcohol (and the list is extensive) are of course responsible for their drinking; however, I argue that the ethos of sport plays a significant and problematic role in such incidents. Furthermore, as I argued in the previous chapter, the visible use of alcohol in sport plays a significant role in the normalization of alcohol use more broadly.

In the preceding chapter, I outlined how the alcohol industry has a vested interest in promoting its product and cultivating a mutually beneficial relationship with sport. I argued that the promotion and marketing of alcohol in general, and through sport in particular, contributes to the normalization of this toxic and potentially harmful substance. The consumption of alcohol is woven into the ethos of sport. This is perhaps an over-generalization and I accept that there will be significant variation between sports and between groups within sport with respect to how alcohol is used and viewed, but in our most visible and popular sports (usually, but not exclusively, male team sport), alcohol continues to feature in a number of problematic ways, not least the high-profile drunken exploits of some of our most prominent athletes.

Ethos

Before I introduce evidence of alcohol's place and role in many of our sporting practices, or describe sport's alcohol ethos, it would be prudent to say a little more about what I mean by an ethos in general, and an ethos that is problematic with respect to alcohol in particular. Although we seem to understand the word ethos when used to express an idea like 'there is a sexist ethos among football fans', the concept can appear vague, slippery, ambiguous or even obscure. An ethos is intangible; it cannot be seen or referred to like a code or set of rules or instructions. It is perhaps better understood in terms of climate, culture, atmosphere, ambience or spirit. McLaughlin (2005: 311–312) argues that:

> At the most general level, an ethos can be regarded as the prevalent or characteristic tone, spirit or sentiment informing an identifiable entity involving human life and interaction (a 'human environment' in the broadest sense) such as a nation, a community, an age, a literature, an institution, an event and so forth. An ethos is evaluative in some sense and is manifested in many aspects of the entity in question and *via* many modes of pervasive influence. The influence of an ethos is seen in shaping of human perceptions, attitudes, beliefs, dispositions and the like in a distinctive way which is implicated in that which is (in some sense) established. Although ethos most commonly refers to something which is experienced, an 'intended' ethos as well as an 'experienced' ethos can be pointed to in the case of an ethos which is deliberately shaped or stipulated.

McLaughlin's account of ethos is rich and complex and there is an obvious *prima facie* resonance for a culture's drinking habits. 'Alcohol ethos' identifies or picks out the 'tone' of a particular practice community with respect to alcohol. An alcohol ethos might be pro-alcohol, in that alcohol and its consumption is actively encouraged. An ethos might be alcohol-tolerant, where alcohol is neither particularly encouraged nor discouraged, or it might be alcohol-intolerant, whereby alcohol is actively discouraged or shunned. The ethos might vary according to age, gender, race, ethnicity, country and sport.

McLaughlin (2005) argues that there can be both an 'intended' ethos and an 'experienced' ethos. The intended ethos is aspirational or normative in the sense that it is a climate or atmosphere that one would like, or feel ought, to pervade a given social practice or context. It might be the 'tone' that the 'powers that be' or the institution or the media aspire to, a set of values that they (leaders, administrators, managers) espouse and encourage among the practice community. Such aspiration may or may not be ethically justifiable, but they are minimally about what is desired. The experienced ethos describes the reality of the prevailing culture of a given practice community. It is the *actual* tone or spirit and is taken for granted and arises spontaneously. The experienced ethos need not be related to the intended ethos in any meaningful way. Where alcohol is concerned, certain members of the practice community (sponsors, governing bodies, player's associations, journalists and coaches) might espouse or aspire towards an ethos characterized as 'professional' (whatever that might mean) in relation to alcohol. The message is unequivocal, that there should be no behaviour involving alcohol (or otherwise) which reflects badly on the sport. The experienced ethos might differ significantly where the use of alcohol is encouraged, particularly on certain occasions such as pre-/post-season tours, celebrations and so forth. According to Vamplew (2005) there are many contradictory practices and attitudes within professional sport when it comes to alcohol consumption. Although there is likely to be universal agreement that letting alcohol interfere with important performances or reputations is bad, in other contexts attitudes might be varied and contradictory. On the one hand, there is the 'professional' attitude espoused by managers and coaches like Arsène Wenger, the coach of Arsenal FC, that alcohol is anathema to elite football players, and former England football team manager, Sven-Göran Eriksson, who stated that drinking alcohol was incompatible with representing your country. On the other hand, it is clear that despite the strong message given by such managers, some players continue to engage in heavy drinking.[1] Other managers continue to allow or turn a blind eye to heavy drinking in the service of team bonding, celebration or stress relief, on the condition that it does not threaten performance or reputation. Vamplew (2005: 406) argues that: 'Players know that drinking alcohol might adversely affect their performance yet they find that their employers are tolerant of a drinking culture . . .'.

A fundamentally important aspect of the experienced ethos is that it is *generative* of individual and collective behaviour, a fact particularly pertinent in terms of drinking practices. According to McLaughlin (2005: 134), the ethos shapes behaviour 'in an indirect and sometimes non-transparent and even unconscious way'. The intended ethos might not have a generative force because it does not resonate or appeal to the practice community, or goes against the grain. It is possible, but difficult, to bring an experienced ethos in line with an intended ethos. This requires significant changes in habits, routine behaviour and attitudes and may take a long time.

Many sociologists of sport turn to Bourdieu (1990) and his concept of *habitus* for a theoretical framework to discuss what I am calling an ethos. Bourdieu argues that social practices such as sport are characterized by a system of rules (explicit and tacit), practical conventions, expectations and ideas, which are both definitive and generative. They are definitive in the sense that these distinctive patterns of social conduct characterize the practice; being a professional athlete involves more than being paid to play – it carries a set of expectations about appearance, socioeconomic status, physical identity and so on. The patterns of social conduct are generative because they motivate or create the action or conduct that embodies the conventions. This happens through initiation, role modelling, creating aspirations and tacit and explicit instruction. Habitus, according to Bourdieu (1990: 53), is a:

> . . . system of durable, transposable dispositions, structured structures predisposed to function as structuring structures, that is, as principles which generate and organize practices and representations that can be objectively adapted to their outcomes without presupposing a conscious aiming at ends or an express mastery of the operations necessary in order to attain them. Objectively regulated and regular without being in any way the product of obedience to rules, they can be collectively orchestrated without being the product of the organizing action of a conductor.

The habitus extends to aspects of the practice beyond the field of play. It does incorporate the important technical and tactical aspects of professional sport, but also covers social conventions, habits, expectations and moral standards. Habitus is therefore generative of both instrumental goal-directed sporting behaviour, and also of patterns of social and moral behaviour, including recreational habits, attitudes towards alcohol, drugs, gambling and women. Dunning and Waddington (2003: 356) describe an ethos of sport which characterized the 'Old Boys' football and cricket teams in Britain after the Second World War. They argue that players were:

> . . . socialized into an acceptance that it is 'manly', not only to play physical contact sports such as football and painful, physically dangerous sports such as cricket, but also to drink beer and to be able to 'hold your ale', that is to drink copious quantities of alcoholic beverages after matches without becoming visibly drunk and losing control.

The habitus described here is recognizable to a greater or lesser extent today. A habitus or ethos is not static or unchanging, but evolves as each new practitioner and each new epoch leaves its mark on the practice. Whatever the ethos amounts to at any given time, however, plays a crucial role in shaping the behaviour, attitudes and values of its members.

Learnt behaviour

So how does the ethos affect the individual drinking habits of players or athletes? One important way we learn particular habits and behaviour is by copying or modelling the behaviour of others around us. According to Bandura (1971: 5): 'Most of the behaviours that people display are learned, either deliberately or inadvertently, through the influence of example'. Not all models (exemplars) are equally effective, and those 'who have high status, prestige, and power are much more effective in evoking matching behaviour in observers than models of low standing' (Bandura 1971: 18). In any particular ethos, if certain behaviours or attitudes are not only modelled, but endorsed or rewarded, particularly by high-status individuals within a particular culture/community, then that behaviour or attitude is more likely to be adopted by other members of the community. Drinking behaviour is a paradigm example. If drinking and being able to 'hold your ale' is accepted, celebrated or 'cool', this will be embodied in the characters of certain individuals and the ethos itself. Those concerned with the health of the population have long studied what influences drinking behaviour with a view to developing effective policies and strategies to reduce consumption levels. Evidence shows that the drinking habits of peer groups and significant others have considerable influence on children and young people, particularly as they transition into adulthood and start to drink. Sussman and Arnett (2014: 147) argue that this period is characterized by risk-taking and 'various substance and behavioural addictions are most likely to be realized during this period'. In many cultures, being able and allowed to drink is a significant marker for adulthood and is often tolerated. The British Medical Association recognizes the key role of 'pro-alcohol' habits (ethos), arguing that:[2]

> The more common and acceptable young people think drinking is, both in society as a whole and among their peers, the more likely they are to be a drinker and the greater quantities of alcohol they are likely to consume.

The alcohol ethos in general, and the alcohol ethos in certain social practices like sport, is crucial in shaping drinking habits. A pro-alcohol ethos gives the impression that drinking alcohol is normal, adult, cool and masculine, and that abstaining is somehow abnormal, boring, weak or feminine. Again, we have to recognize that there will be variation within and between sports in terms of age, gender, race, ethnicity, level, cultural context and so on. In a study with a student population, Orford et al. (2004) identified more specifically some of the social factors that influenced drinking, including social interaction, 'having a laugh' and self-confidence. They found that:

> ... heavy drinkers would receive more encouragement to drink from important people in their lives than light drinkers, suggesting that not only are heavy drinkers' social networks drinking more, but that their opinions and behaviours are directly influencing their fellow students . . . . (Orford et al. 2004: 418)

Wynn et al. (1997) argue that social pressure to use alcohol, including peer pressure, are among the most important factors in the misuse of alcohol among the younger population. They argue that, like adults, there may be a number of motives for adolescent drinking, for example, to relieve tension or to increase self-confidence (essentially, as mentioned in Chapter 1, alcohol changes the mood in some way), 'but without a social context [ethos] that permits and promotes drinking, adolescents are unlikely to drink' (Wynn et al. 1997: 390). Spijkerman et al. (2007: 8) report that research on adolescent drinkers suggests that one of the factors why adolescents start drinking is in order to cultivate characteristics 'associated with the type of person who performs these types of behaviour', in other words, because they aspire to the image or appearance of the role model or 'prototypes'.

As I have mentioned, it is inaccurate to universalize when talking about an ethos of sport or a pro-alcohol ethos in sport. It is not my intention to offer here a detailed descriptive or nuanced account of any particular sporting sub-culture, each with its own unique alcohol ethos. What follows, however, is a brief overview of three broad categories of sport; namely, youth and community sport, college or varsity sport (both in the USA and the UK, although I recognize that these are very different practices) and elite professional sport. The two former categories have been widely researched with respect to alcohol consumption, whereas insights into alcohol use in the latter comes largely via anecdotes, the media, biographies and autobiographies. What I aim to show is that all, to a greater or lesser extent, can be said to have an ethos where the use and misuse of alcohol is fairly common and valued.

Youth and community sport

For many, both their early and continued experience with sport is at a local club. Some graduate from these clubs to greater things, but many start and finish their sporting career at their local football, rugby, tennis or swimming club. They not only provide opportunities to play sport, but they are a focus of social interaction and community intercourse. As such, according to Duff and Munro (2007: 1992), community sports clubs provide a significant positive role in 'providing and developing social connections and civic participation sporting clubs contribute to the emotional, social and mental health of the community'. The virtues of such community sports clubs are not in doubt, and the efforts of parents, volunteers and coaches who run them provide children and adults with a wide range of valuable experiences and opportunities beyond the sporting contest. These include charitable fundraising events, trips abroad and engagement with community projects, among other things. Despite these virtues, Duff and Munro (2007: 1992) argue that 'sports clubs in Australia are notorious for the rates of unregulated, high-risk drinking'. Worryingly, it seems that such venues are also more likely to serve underage drinkers than others venues where alcohol is sold. In the UK, a young athlete's first pint is often at the rugby or football club before their 18th birthday. It is a 'coming of age' or transitional ritual. Crundall (2012: 97) argues that excessive drinking is commonplace in community sports clubs characterized by 'ritual binge-drinking, performances being rewarded with alcohol, alcohol-fuelled end-of-season trips, drinking competitions, and "all-you-can-drink" functions' and 'alcohol is reinforced as integral to club participation, relaxation and the celebration or commiseration of wins and loses'. Black et al. (1999: 201) found that non-elite sportsmen were more likely to drink excessively 'when socializing with sporting team mates compared to drinking on social occasions with other groups'. A recreational rugby player died from alcohol poisoning on his stag night (bachelor party) after he and his friends engaged in a drinking game known as 'the dentist's chair'. Perhaps inspired by the antics of Paul Gascoigne and the England football team in Hong Kong in 1996, Paul Tobutt had strong spirits poured down his throat while sitting in a dentist's chair in a bar in Spain. He died as a direct consequence of this dangerous drinking game, encouraged and cheered on by his 'friends' and teammates.[3]

Research shows that it is not only club or community sport that poses a risk. Denham (2011: 364) found that both male and female athletes at the adolescent level in the USA 'tend to consume alcohol more often than their peers', and Eccles and Barber (1999) similarly found that participation in team sports was linked to high rates of involvement in drinking alcohol among pupils, again in the USA. It appears that involvement in secondary school sport in the UK is also likely to influence drinking. Davies and Foxall (2011) suggest that: 'UK male teenage athletes [aged 14 and 15 years] appear to have a higher level of involvement with alcohol, particularly in terms of excess consumption, than do their non-athletic peers'. The drinking is not only restricted to teenagers. Teachers and coaches sometimes exemplify poor behaviour with alcohol. Recently on a UK secondary school sport's trip to Barcelona, the teachers who were looking after the children got involved in a drunken brawl.[4] Peck et al. (2008: 70), however, found that: 'Participating in sports is not necessarily a risk or protective factor for alcohol use'. Nevertheless, in a meta-analysis, Diehl et al. (2012: 201) concluded that: 'Although report of risky behaviors varied across studies, we observed overall that studies tend to report higher alcohol use ... in (high-involved) athletes'.[5] There were differences between types of sport, the demographics of participants within sport and the level of sport played.

The patterns of drinking among adolescents reflect a general pattern of difference in drinking along certain demographic lines. Generally speaking, the problem was worse among white males and females, with males drinking more, and more often, than females. Sometimes there was an ethos within an ethos, where 'team members would cluster by race and ethnicity within the larger team environment' (Denham 2011: 372). As might be expected, Denham (2011) also found differences according to the nature of the sport – in particular team versus individual – and the demands of the sport itself.

The college experience

In many cultures, student or varsity sport has a reputation for excessive alcohol consumption and its concomitant problems, and, from continuing personal experience, it is well deserved. Brenner and Swanik (2007: 270) found that 75% of the USA college athletes surveyed reported being high-risk drinkers and 44% were frequent high-risk drinkers, with the problem worse among team sport athletes. They concluded that 'heavy alcohol use by college athletes is very much a social phenomenon'. Ford (2007: 1368) argues that college students involved in athletics 'are more likely to engage in a wide range of risky behaviour than non-athletes are' which includes binge drinking and heavy alcohol use. In particular, athletes report more extreme styles of alcohol consumption, binge drink at higher rates, are more likely to binge when they drink and get drunk more often. Borsari and Carey (2001) argue that college students use alcohol to conform to group expectations of behaviour and to avoid negative evaluations from peers (ethos). Failure to conform to group norms, by not using alcohol, may result in rejection by peers and social isolation. Green et al. (2014: 424) found that participation in organized sports at college is positively associated with binge drinking. They found that the relationship holds true 'across racial and sex division' and continues after engagement with sport has ended. Kerr et al. (2014) found that former college athletes were more likely to be dependent on alcohol than the general population in the USA. Martens et al. (2006) found that there were differences between sports and, perhaps surprisingly, found that swimmers and divers reported the highest level of alcohol consumption. Of course student drinking extends beyond athletes and alcohol causes many problems on campuses. Boston University has made public the statistics on alcohol-related problems in order to try and reduce excessive alcohol use, primarily to curb the incidence of sexual violence.[6]

O'Brien et al. (2008: 663) found that hazardous drinking and frequent drinking was high for both male and female university athletes in New Zealand. Their results seem to buck the trend of a gender difference. 'We found that there were no significant differences between male and female university sportspeople's level of drinking, dependence symptoms or negative consequences . . .'. McDonald and Sylvester (2014) found that learning to drink was an important element of university sports clubs in Japan and coming to know how to drink (an important part of Japanese social interaction) involved negotiating sports clubs drinking parties. Partington et al. (2013: 344) found that in the UK:

> . . . members of university sport groups were found to consume greater quantities of alcohol, to be more at risk for alcohol-related harm, to drink more frequently, to consume greater quantities of alcohol on a typical drinking occasion, and to engage in heavy episodic drinking more regularly than students not engaged in university sports.

Zhou et al. (2014) found that 89% of the UK-based sporting students they surveyed reported hazardous drinking levels with women being slightly more likely to have engaged than men. They found that drinking for team cohesion was the strongest predictor of hazardous drinking.

Evidence therefore points to the fact that the sports culture, often referred to as a 'jock culture', at universities, is characterized by a potentially problematic or risky alcohol ethos. Sparkes et al. (2007) sought to interrogate the university sport experience in the UK further, and found that alcohol consumption and associated drinking practices played a central role in the maintenance of embodied jock culture at UK universities. Using Bourdieu's (1990) notion of physical capital, a means of attaining and/or exchanging value in social settings or cultural contexts like sporting teams, they found that the ability or willingness to consume large amounts of alcohol was seen as important for fitting into, and gaining status and prestige within, the team habitus. They proposed 'twelve commandments', which in Bourdieu's terms served as 'structured and structuring practical logic in operation' (Sparkes et al. 2007: 304). The consumption of alcohol featured in four of these commandments, namely, 'be committed to the social life', 'excessive alcohol consumption and associated behaviours are obligatory', 'attend socials regularly' and 'attend post-match drinking sessions'. Excessive alcohol consumption goes as far as vomiting and collapse, but is also associated with behaviours such as participation in drinking games and the associated forfeits, which may include stripping naked and performing a range of other problematic challenges. Sparkes et al. (2007: 314) argued that students can:

> . . . use their bodies to good effect in other arenas associated with culture to gain acceptance. For example, consuming an excessive amount of alcohol

and engaging in associated behaviours is as much an embodied performance as playing as sport and the physical capital involved in the former can also be exchanged for social capital.

Clayton (2012) provides further insight into a specific and potentially problematic element of sporting culture in general, and student jock culture in particular; namely, initiation ceremonies or 'hazing'. Hazing involves putting new recruits through ritualistic tests 'that involve physical abuse, psychological damage, and sexual humiliation' (Anderson et al. 2012: 427–428). On such occasions, newcomers to a team or club are forced to undertake humiliating and risky behaviours. Anderson et al. (2012), during a longitudinal ethnographic study of hazing at a UK university, found four token types of hazing ritual, namely, physical acts of violence, anti-social behaviour, excessive alcohol consumption and same-sex sexual activities (the latter decreased in number over the period of the study). Hazing occasions are characterized by 'the familiar discourse of macho laddism, the competitiveness, the nudity, the heavy drinking and the pursuit of girls . . .' (Clayton 2012: 215). Such occasions can get out of hand and have serious consequences including fatalities.[7] On 20 September 2010, members of the University of Gloucestershire's men's rugby and football clubs committed lewd sex acts on public transport as part of a drunken initiation ceremony. The judge at their hearing condemned the bullying and humiliating sport club culture which encouraged drunken bad behaviour.[8] There are plenty of other disturbing examples of hazing and its negative consequences in university sport, and although Clayton (2012) and others are primarily referring to male sport, women and girls are increasingly engaging in risky drinking behaviour during initiation or hazing ceremonies. Anecdotal evidence from my institution, Cardiff Metropolitan University, suggests that girls' team sports like field hockey are particularly debauched in terms of obligatory post-match heavy drinking and initiation ceremonies.

The professional/elite experience

According to Vamplew (2005: 396), the alcohol consumption of athletes reflects the patterns in society in general, and alcohol is used 'to relieve stress and for convivial recreational purposes'. Despite the problems associated with alcohol in general, and for sports participation in particular, Vamplew (2005: 397) argues that 'teetotallers are probably in the minority in British sport'. It is perhaps the case that young physically fit athletes see themselves as immune from the addictive and adverse effects of alcohol. There is perhaps some justification for such beliefs because athletes, at least in certain sports, have been able to excel without eliminating alcohol from their lives.[9] In fact, there are a number of athletes who achieved excellent performance levels despite being 'abusers' of alcohol. Ray Parlour, the former Arsenal football player, recounts how he and fellow players used to drink heavily on occasions and were very successful despite the drink culture. The culture changed when Arsène Wenger took over as manager and sought to change the drinking ethos at the club.[10]

Studies into the drinking ethos of professional sports teams are not as easy to come by as those for amateur or college sports for a host of reasons. Nevertheless, anecdotal evidence, off-the-record conversations with professional athletes, biographies, autobiographies, the press, social media sites like Twitter and Facebook, and personal experience provide some insight into the role alcohol plays in the lives of professional athletes and into the alcohol ethos of some sports. Given the level of performance demanded from elite athletes and alcohol's potential threat to that performance, it seems that, for most, abstention or at least careful moderation is chosen when performance might be threatened. Nevertheless, if the threat to performance is taken out of the equation, for example, at the end of an important tournament or when there is ample time to recover before the next tournament, an alcohol binge continues to be 'part and parcel' of the professional sporting ethos.[11] At the London 2012 Olympic village the USA team had two sponsored beer halls: Budweiser House and Heineken House.[12]

A particularly prominent rugby union player in the UK, through his actions and written recollections, provides an insight into the alcohol ethos in professional rugby. In his autobiography, Gavin Henson, a former Welsh rugby union international, and a somewhat controversial figure, recalls his initiation into team bonding as a young professional rugby union player in south Wales:

> Rugby and drinking have always gone together, but I've never found it an easy mix. That summer of 2000 when I joined Swansea, John Plumtree decided we needed a 'bonding session' to pull the whole squad together before the season started. The bonding consisted of a drinking marathon down the sea-front from St Helen's in Mumbles, a village where the pubs and bars are all within easy staggering distances of each other. Dean Thomas, the Swansea flanker at the time and a hard player, grabbed me and insisted I start off matching him round for round. I was even more of a hopeless drinker then than I am now and it wasn't long before I was completely leathered. I may have 'bonded' with Dean but I don't remember much about it. Too smashed to go on, I rang my parents and my father drove 30 miles from Bridgend to come and pick me up. I spewed all the way home, but Dad didn't seem too shocked. I think he understood. (Henson 2005: 102)

Later in his career, in 2005, at the end of a very successful Six Nations Championship in which he (Gavin Henson) had excelled and scored some crucial points, his team's sponsors at the time, S.A. Brain (discussed in Chapter 2), organized a celebration for the Wales team. The anecdote illustrates the alcohol ethos of this particular team at this particular time very clearly:

> I met up with Charlotte [his girlfriend] at the after-match dinner before all the players, plus wives and girlfriends, went to a function laid on by Brains, the brewers who had become our shirt sponsor. Needless to say, the beer was on them. We enjoyed a great night and it felt good to be together in celebration with the same guys I had been alongside for many weeks. Like the rest of

Cardiff, and the rest of Wales, we made sure the party went on long into the night and I eventually made it back to the team hotel about 5 am. The next morning I had hoped to spend recovering from the night before. But after doing all the media interviews there was a call from the team management to be ready to board the bus by noon. It appeared the celebrations were still in full swing. I had a horrible hangover but managed to get my head together after a few bottles of water and limped onto the team bus. I was wrecked. We were driven into the centre of Cardiff and dropped at a bar called The Yard, a pub owned by Brains . . . . Downstairs were punters who looked as if they hadn't been to bed from the night before, but we were ushered upstairs and into another private party . . . . It wasn't long before all the players were playing drinking games to get in the mood and not very long at all before I was completely smashed. This was a players' only deal. No wives. No girlfriends. So it was all a bit macho and a bit excessive to say the least. (Henson 2005: 74–75)

As a result of getting drunk at this session, Henson vandalized the toilets, scuffled with bouncers and generally behaved badly, but escaped arrest. Henson's name would feature frequently in press reports about the drinking and socializing exploits of Welsh rugby union players. One security company which provides security staff (bouncers) for a number of licensed premises in Cardiff decided to ban him because he was often drunk. A spokesperson for the company told the local press that: 'All the door staff are fed up with Gavin Henson because he's an absolute nightmare when he is drinking'.[13] Henson was not out alone and was often with other members of the Wales rugby union team celebrating (or drowning their sorrows) after an important game. A journalist close to the Welsh rugby union team indicated to me that the perceived problem (from within the team) with Gavin Henson was that he could not 'hold his drink'. In other words, the culture of drinking heavily in pubs to celebrate is not problematic; the problem lies with certain individuals unable to cope with the 'expected' volume of alcohol and behaving inappropriately as a consequence. Henson made the headlines on a number of other occasions for his drinking, including urinating on a train and being drunk on a 7 am flight from Glasgow back to Cardiff after his team had played a match there the night before.[14]

Andy Powell, another Welsh rugby union player, was arrested in the early hours of the morning (5.40 am) following an international match with Scotland in 2010. He is alleged to have stolen a golf cart from the team hotel in a golf resort while drunk, and driven it on public roads including a motorway. The police charged him with 'driving a mechanically propelled vehicle whilst unfit through drink'. He was dropped from the Welsh squad for the remainder of the Six Nations Championship on the grounds that his behaviour was contrary to the squad's code of conduct.[15] The incident happened after the Welsh team beat Scotland in spectacular fashion and it seems that the team were given license to 'celebrate'. This involved heavy drinking by players and coaches alike. We do not know the full details of what happened, but I am making the following assumption; that Powell's drinking, although not his behaviour when drunk, was in line with the ethos of celebrating victories by drinking heavily. In other words, getting extremely drunk was an expectation or perhaps an obligation (as indicated by Henson above) under those circumstances. The response of the public to Powell's antics suggests that not only is drinking part of the ethos, but a certain level of 'high jinks' is to be expected. A Facebook page was started entitled Andy Powell Appreciation Society for Driving a Golf Cart Buggy on the M4, celebrating or 'valorizing' his antics to the extent that it received more than 100 000 'likes'.[16]

Rugby union is a sport that has always been strongly associated with a drink culture at all levels. In an interview on BBC television's Breakfast programme, Matt Dawson, a winner of the Rugby World Cup with England, provided an insight into the drinking culture of professional rugby. He opined that:[17]

> . . . binge drinking, there is a culture of rugby players enjoying a drink, and I say long may that continue because rugby is a magnificent game on and off the field and it does involve having a good time and having a couple of beers, but it's all about control.

A former teammate of Dawson, Martin Johnson, was the coach of the English rugby union team at the 2011 Rugby World Cup. The team experienced a below-par performance, exiting the tournament prematurely. The British media were quick to criticize the performance of the English team, and the alcohol ethos featured prominently in headlines and column inches in both tabloid and broadsheet newspapers as well as on television, radio and the internet. A number of England players, including the captain, Mike Tindall, had gone out drinking during the tournament to a bar which had a 'dwarf throwing' competition. Photos of the players, including one of Tindall with a young woman (not his wife, Zara Phillips), made it into the tabloids. The press on this occasion seemed to take a hard line. Professional athletes representing their country at an international competition should not be consuming alcohol in public clubs and bars where their behaviour would inevitably be scrutinized. The Welsh rugby union team, on the other hand, found themselves in a position as exemplar professionals with Sam Warburton, a young, self-confessed tee-totaller, as captain. Their fitness and performance standards along with their exemplary conduct off the field made the Welsh the paragons in comparison to the England team and their captain. Warren Gatland, the Welsh team coach, felt the need to temper the media-generated 'goody two shoes' image of his team. He was quick to reject the idea that there was an 'alcohol ban' within the squad and insisted that his team were 'no monks'. There may have been many reasons for this. Members of his own squad had far from exemplary records in terms of public drunkenness prior to the tournament, and he wanted to avoid any potential hypocrisy or be seen to stand in judgement on others.[18] He was also keen to diffuse any additional pressure that being cast as exemplary professionals might have on his young squad.[19] Martin Johnson did not see fit to punish the actions of his team's captain at the time, because presumably they were in line with the experienced ethos (having a few drinks). In light of the media scrutiny which followed, however, the governing body, Rugby Football

Union, subsequently fined Tindall £25 000 and removed him from the elite play-ing squad. Such behaviour was clearly not part of the intended ethos. Part of the punishment was for misleading the England management team, but the tariff was reduced on appeal to £15 000. His partly successful appeal was based on the fact that he did not intentionally mislead the management team, presumably because of the effects of alcohol: *he just could not remember events clearly!*

There are countless other incidents and insights into the alcohol ethos of pro-fessional rugby (both union and league) in the UK, Australia, New Zealand and elsewhere. A number of players from the professional rugby union side, Newport Gwent Dragons, in the UK, were involved in a fight outside a pub celebrating the end of the season,[20] and Gavin Henson was involved yet again in some trouble in a pub with his teammates while at Bath RFC.[21] Another name which features prominently is the English player, Danny Cipriani. His latest of a long line of alcohol-related misfortunes occurred during a team bonding event. His team, Sale Sharks, were on a fancy dress pub crawl in Leeds, in 2013, when Cipriani was hit by a bus and had to be taken to hospital.[22] In November 2013, Australia's national rugby union team banned six players during their visit to the UK and Ireland. Their coach, Ewan McKenzie, took the action because 'a group of players made the decision to stay out late and consume inappropriate levels of alcohol', and nine further players were also disciplined.[23] Aaron Cruden was banned by the New Zealand All Blacks for two games after he missed the team's flight to Argentina following a night out drinking.[24]

Professional football (soccer), particularly in the UK, also seems to have a culture of drinking. The autobiographies of retried players are rife with stories of alcohol-fuelled parties, pre-season tours and incidents, many of which came to the public's attention. Stories of players out partying, enjoying the trappings of their millionaire lifestyles, are common. Some players head to Las Vegas, Dubai, Miami or other party destinations when time permits at the end of the season to indulge in champagne, party with glamour models and take full advantage of the hedonistic opportunities available for young famous millionaires. Thousands of pounds are spent on hotels, expensive alcohol, exclusive clubs and parties.[25]

Players drink, sometimes with, sometimes without, the blessing of their clubs or coaches. Roy Keane recently revealed that drinking was his 'hobby' at Manchester United FC, and that he was involved in a fight with a team-mate during a drinking session on a pre-season tour. Craig Bellamy similarly assaulted a teammate with a golf club during a tour with Liverpool FC. Such stories appear in the tabloids and on social media on a weekly basis. *The Sun*, a UK tabloid newspaper, reported that Harry Redknapp, Tottenham Hotspur FC manager, would not allow his players to 'drown their sorrows' following their FA Cup final defeat.[26] He was quoted as saying: '. . . I would say to any player: Why do you need to booze?', a sentiment lost on some of his players including Ledley King,[27] Peter Crouch and Jonathan Woodgate, all of whom have since made headlines in the tabloid newspapers for their drunken exploits.[28] More troubling for Harry Redknapp was his players' covert Christmas party, despite him expressly forbidding such an event a few days earlier.[29] The examples of

Christmas parties, celebrations, foreign trips and nights out ending up in the newspapers are legion. Players staying out late, getting into fights and engaging in inappropriate and sometimes illegal sexual activity feature routinely on the front and sport pages of British newspapers. A recent example again featured Harry Redknapp and the Premier League club Queens Park Rangers, a team he managed at the time. It is *alleged* that a mid-season club training trip to Dubai in 2013 turned into a 'stag party' with un-sanctioned all-night drinking and ill-discipline.[30]

A common consequence of the drinking of professional footballers is that there are often female victims or alleged victims. Again, there are countless examples of players involved in inappropriate sexual behaviour when drunk, such as the four Brighton and Hove Albion FC players who had been drinking to celebrate a cup win in 2011. They were charged with sexually assaulting a sleeping teenager in a hotel room.[31] Furthermore, seven players from Crewe Alexandra FC were arrested over an alleged sexual assault in 2013.[32]

One particularly worrying aspect of the drinking ethos in sport in the UK seems to be the attitude towards driving under the influence of alcohol. There are a number of convictions among high-profile professional athletes, particularly among male rugby, cricket and football players, ex-players and managers. Although examples are numerous, a few are particularly noteworthy. The first is the example of Luke McCormick, a professional goalkeeper in England who tragically killed two young children while driving under the influence of alcohol. Rio Ferdinand, a recent former England football team captain, was convicted of driving under the influence of alcohol, and Mike Tindall, a recent former England rugby union team captain, has twice been convicted of driving under the influence of alcohol. Steve Kean was convicted of driving under the influence of alcohol while manager of Blackburn Rovers FC. Such convictions do not seem at odds with the professional ethos in the UK, and such crimes are rarely held against players or managers when it comes to internal discipline or recruitment.

There is a similar alcohol culture in certain professional North American sports, particularly, but not exclusively, male team sports. Theo Fleury, the Canadian ice hockey player, recalls a number of habits and traditions:

> Every single night after a game, we'd go out and get wasted. Almost everybody on the whole team. We were always together, drinking and partying. There was a bar called the Green Parrot across from the rink. We used to go there all the time. (Fleury 2009: 53)

> As I said before, drinking in the NHL happened. It was like any group of college kids or twenty somethings. Getting pissed was a great way to bond. Most of the coaches left you alone as long as you produced. I showed up many times in the morning completely annihilated. I hadn't even gone home yet. How did I perform? Awesome. Sometimes I would come in a little slow, hungover from the night before, but I dealt with it by drinking a coffee and smoking three or four cigarettes. I was having a full-body orgasm. Money,

fame and chicks. I made the most of it. What was I going to do? Slow down, stay home every night and watch TV? Forget it. (Fleury 2009: 63)

Josh Hamilton describes his return to baseball after expulsion because of his crack cocaine addiction. As a 'newcomer' to the team there were certain traditions and practices that could potentially compromise his recovery:

> Being a rookie is difficult enough, but being a different kind of rookie made it that much harder. I am not a confrontational person by nature, and rookies are supposed to be subservient in the baseball culture, but there were times when the baseball culture and my well-being came into conflict . . . . Most of the traditions are meant to be in good fun, and I played along just fine. But one rookie duty is to carry the beer on road trips. Alcohol is a big part of the culture in baseball, although recent events – especially the tragedy of pitcher Josh Hancock's death in St Louis – have forced baseball to take a closer look at the intelligence of letting players use the clubhouse as a bar after games . . . . But before the first road trip of my rookie season, I declined when I was asked – or rather told – to carry the beer by one of the veterans. (Hamilton 2008: 226)

The examples I have listed in all the categories above are primarily male team sports. However, there is clear evidence that the ethos of drinking is neither an exclusively team sport (boxing, tennis, golf and cycling at the elite level have had a number of heavy drinkers, if the autobiographical testimony of athletes like Sugar Ray Leonard, Mike Tyson, Ricky Hatton, Andre Agassi, John McEnroe, John Daly and Bradley Wiggins are representative) nor a male preserve. Women have embraced many aspects of the alcohol ethos, which includes heavy drinking, initiation ceremonies and singing crude songs, both in traditionally masculine sports such as football (soccer), rugby (union and league) and ice hockey, and in more traditionally feminine team sports such as field hockey.[33] In other words, women (in certain sports) are embracing fully both the positive and negative elements of traditional jock culture. According to Collins and Vamplew (2002: 101): 'Many women who play rugby union also appear to have adopted this cultural attitude and aspire to emulate the male members of their club in drinking feats'. The Canadian women's national ice hockey team celebrated their gold medal victory at the Vancouver Winter Olympics in 2010 in a manner that aped their male counterparts' celebration rituals. The team 'sat at centre ice, smoked cigars, drank cans of Molson Canadian beer and gulped champagne' and engaged in boisterous celebrations which included driving the 'Zamboni' (ice-resurfacing machine) around the rink (Edwards et al. 2013: 682). Kelly Smith describes her drinking, which eventually became alcoholic, within the team culture of women's football while playing in the college system in the USA. There were plenty of opportunities to party and she describes herself as one of the 'big drinkers in her team' (Smith 2012: 35).

Alcohol, masculinity and a macho ethos

The ethos described above of course involves far more than alcohol consumption. As mentioned there are a host of other ideas, beliefs, habits and traditions inextricably linked with the use of alcohol. De Visser and Smith (2007) argue that alcohol consumption is important in the formation and portrayal of masculine identity. Similarly, sport has been a touchstone of masculinity and it is perhaps not surprising that sport and alcohol are close companions. In the sporting context, particularly in traditional team games, being able to drink or being able to hold one's drink is very much part of the cultivation of masculinity and masculine identity (Dunning and Waddington 2003). Although there are many forms of masculinity, the dominant masculine discourse or hegemonic masculinity is 'characterised by physical and emotional toughness, risk taking, predatory heterosexuality, being a breadwinner . . .' (De Visser and Smith 2007: 597). In sport, at its worst the form of masculinity has been described by Davis (2012: 5) as the 'fag end of masculinity' and is characterized by, among other things, sexism, homophobia, power, misogyny and the consumption of alcohol (often exemplified in rituals like initiations or fan behaviour).

In other words, it is 'macho' not just to drink, but to be able to hold your drink, and a bad drinker's masculine credentials are often questioned, often in sexist and homophobic terms such as 'poof', 'pussy', 'girl', 'light weight' and so on (Black et al. 1999). Given that different behaviours contribute to masculine identity, De Visser and Smith (2007) argue that a lack of competence in one, perhaps not being a good athlete, or not being successful with women, could be compensated for by competence in relation to another, such as drinking. Within a given sport's team, drinking prowess is a form of 'cultural capital' and may compensate for lack of sporting or physical prowess. Being the drinker, the entertainer or the risk-taker carries some kudos within a team environment, and such an individual might play a crucial role in instigating and conducting other behaviours and rituals which define the masculine narrative of the habitus or ethos.

There has been growing concern in general, and in the sporting context in particular, that women and girls are embracing some of the worst excesses of masculinity, with the nadir being behaviour while drinking alcohol. The term 'ladette' was coined (at least in the UK) to describe, or perhaps criticize, young women who manifest certain traditionally male behaviours including drinking and sexual promiscuity. Sport is a context where ladette behaviour finds a comfortable and perhaps even extreme form, and according to Edwards et al. (2013: 690) 'ladettes challenge normative ideas of acceptable femininity by being too masculine'. Notwithstanding the significant complexities surrounding contemporary masculinity and femininity in sport, the point here is that masculinity plays a key role in the ethos of excessive drinking in sport for both men and women and it is the consequence of excessive drinking that is my primary concern.

What's the harm?

In Chapter 1 I outlined some of the harms associated with excessive drinking. Such harms, of course, may befall those drinking excessively in the sports context, but some are particularly prominent given the ethos described above. An ethos that valorizes the consumption of alcohol at dangerous levels, and in some cases enforces such consumption through initiation ceremonies, drinking games and so forth, is particularly dangerous and repugnant. A whole host of chronic and acute harms from the toxic effects of alcohol result as a consequence of heavy episodic drinking (binge drinking). Harms to others include violence, sexual impropriety, sexual assault, accidents, driving under the influence and the risk of bringing one's employer and profession into disrepute. Alcohol, young fit athletes and a macho culture are a potent recipe for problems. Many athletes have been involved in violent incidents when drunk. Recent examples include Australian cricketer, David Warner, who attacked the English cricketer, Joe Root, in a late-night incident in a bar during the Ashes Test cricket series in 2013. He had been drinking vodka and Jägerbombs in drinking sessions with teammates.[34] Drunken athletes involved in problematic sexual activity is a common issue in many cultures. Countless high-profile athletes have been embroiled in accusations of rape and sexual assault.[35] We have seen how, in some cases, the experienced ethos of sport encourages and celebrates both risky drinking and risk-taking when drunk. The ethos not only normalizes excessive drinking, but also cultivates a misaligned sense of safe and sensible levels of alcohol consumption, even if no further problems arise. Although athletes are fit, they are not immune to the effects alcohol may have on their bodies. Even 'moderate' post-game or post-training drinking can be excessive in comparison to UK health recommendations. Tony Adams recalls drinking up to 20 pints of Guinness and more when he went out with teammates (Adams 1998: 203). What is certain is that a 'few beers' means more than 2 pints. Moreover, the 'feast or famine' that characterizes athletes' drinking, particularly elite athletes, is considered to be more risky than spreading alcohol intake evenly.

The power of the ethos

In 2014, in the UK, a new craze spread through social media sites, called 'necknominate'. The 'game' involved filming oneself downing an alcoholic drink, posting the film on social media and nominating (or challenging) someone else to do the same. As the craze developed, people were downing bigger, stronger and more dangerous cocktails of alcohol. Inevitably, a number of deaths followed, including a young rugby player who died after drinking 2 pints of gin.[36] In another incident, a 9-year-old girl was hospitalized after she and her friends copied the game after seeing it on Facebook.[37] The game is alleged to have been started by a professional rugby league player. The practice of downing a pint of alcohol quickly (or the old yard of ale or even, in some cases, urine or vomit) to the cheers or encouragement of one's teammates (variations include standing on a chair or being naked) is a staple of post-match drinking culture with the man of the match or in some cases the 'prat (insert any insulting word to describe the worst player) of the match' being compelled to drink as a 'reward' or forfeit. Other occasions like scoring, a birthday, first game and so on might also be an occasion for the ritual. Taking the ritual from the confines of the clubhouse onto the internet caused untold harm. The point here is not so much that the game was borne out of common practice in sports cultures, but that the prevailing ethos/culture/values can have a very powerful influence on how people behave. The power of expectation, the desire to fit in and to copy, and the fear of ridicule for a failure in masculine courage, contributed to countless individuals risking (and sometimes losing) their lives by drinking dangerous levels of alcohol.

At certain times the ethos of certain sports, both experienced and intended, demand that individuals engage in heavy drinking and other related activities such as drinking games. For many, this is experienced as neither a demand nor an obligation, but as volitional and pleasurable (just as some of those who engaged in necknomination, 'nobody forced them to drink'). Of course, individuals have the option to exercise their own agency and make their own choices when it comes to the consumption of alcohol. As we have seen, however, we should not underestimate the power of cultural expectations and peer pressure on individual behaviour. Blum (1994) argues that the community and the exercise of virtues and vices (more of which in next chapter) are linked in a number of significant ways. Virtues and vices can only be learned and nurtured 'within particular forms of social life' and communities (the ethos) provide the content for our moral values, ideals and principles. In other words, an ideal or principle like loyalty or commitment can be understood in the abstract, but it is the community that teaches us what actions count as commitment or instantiate loyalty. It is only 'by living within a complex form of communal life can we learn these particulars' (Blum 1994: 147). Learning to be, and demonstrating one is, a committed member of the team might involve a commitment to organized social activities and drinking practices (Sparkes et al. 2007). Another important way in which a community plays a significant role is by conferring value to certain practices and behaviours. There are some qualities that are only qualities vis-à-vis the particular standards and expectations of a particular community. 'One could not see the quality as virtuous – or even really understand what the quality was – except by being part of the community in question' (Blum 1994: 147). There are certain 'qualities' celebrated within sporting cultures that are unfathomable or, at least, not seen as qualities outside that community or other similar communities. Many have been mentioned already, like the ability to drink lots of alcohol, or being prepared to take risks or fulfil certain dares and challenges as part of ritualized drinking activities. In my experience with rugby clubs, the ability (if that is the right word) or willingness to drink urine or vomit was celebrated, although only a few would ever be willing or stupid enough to do so.

But can an ethos or community really compromise autonomy or shape behaviour in the extreme ways discussed here? There are a few possible responses to such a question. The first is to reiterate the observations already made, that what might appear extreme or unusual to outsiders can be routine and normal to insiders. The second is to refer to evidence that testifies to the power of the situation and its features (for example, peer pressure, expectations and so on) in individual behaviour and action. Over the last half century, evidence from social psychology has increased our understanding of personality and agency and how it interacts with the social environment. Perhaps the most (in)famous studies are the series of experiments conducted by Stanley Milgram. Milgram (1964) designed and conducted experiments to see how far individuals would go in conforming to an authority figure. Subjects who thought they were involved in a learning experiment were asked to administer incremental levels of electric shocks to learners (confederates). His findings shocked the USA as the majority of the subjects administered electric shocks at levels that would have been fatal if they had been real. They seemed to be reluctant or incapable of exercising their autonomy when faced with a specific set of circumstances that demanded obedience. What these and other similar studies show is how individual agency can be influenced or compromised by prevailing situational cues. The data from studies prove that, as individuals we are particularly susceptible to contextual influences, and can make choices we never thought we would, and which we subsequently come to regret. Complying with dominant authority figures, copying the behaviour of others in the group, trying to 'fit in', have all been found by researchers to influence behaviour in various ways (Flanagan 1991: 298–301). This kind of situational pressure is common in a drinking context in general, and in sport in particular. Perhaps one of the most recent and shocking examples of such pressure in the context of drinking is the disturbing actions of a young woman on holiday in the party resort of Magaluf, Ibiza. The 18 year old was encouraged to perform oral sex on 24 male clubbers. The alcohol-fuelled sexualized party atmosphere contributed/ caused the woman to comply with the expectations of the nightclub full of peers. Inevitably, the episode was filmed and came to light through social media. Of course, this young woman has to take some responsibility, but the drinking and party culture and the irresponsible cajoling and promotion of excessive drinking by particular venues and entire resorts play a key role.[38] Exercising a choice not to drink, or to drink moderately, is often greeted with derision and ridicule. There is, at least in the UK, a stock vocabulary used by 'the group' to try and influence behaviour. Expressions like 'light weight', 'jibber' and 'killjoy' are among some of the more polite provocations designed to incite drinking. Goading non-drinkers by questioning their masculinity, sexuality and toughness are par for the course in sport. The alcohol ethos and individuals who 'set the agenda' in terms of expected alcohol consumption will have a powerful and demonstrable influence on certain individuals in particular, and the alcohol ethos in general (positive or negative).

Changing the ethos

If we are committed to avoiding individual incidents of alcohol-related deviance among elite athletes, a key consideration is to address the ethos that teaches, sustains and celebrates excessive alcohol consumption. Many, but not all, of the problems arise because the experienced (and even the intended) ethos of sporting cultures and communities is unhealthy as far as alcohol is concerned because it normalizes the consumption of excessive volumes (in comparison to recommended units) and encourages a host of related rituals and behaviours tied to or made worse by binge drinking. The individual who oversteps the mark is rightly punished for their actions, but unless the ethos is changed the continuous stream of stories about athletes being drunk will endure because they are still being taught that drinking heavily is normal, acceptable and valued. Of course, it is important to address the behaviour of an individual (see Chapters 5, 6 and 7), but the culture and ethos which provide the conditions that allow such individuals to survive and even flourish has to be changed. Flanagan (1991: 313) makes the point in the following way:

> . . . knowledge of the situational factors which in interaction with certain characteristic dispositional configurations result in morally problematic behaviour gives us information which can be exceedingly valuable if we want and are able to put our minds to the project of keeping such situations from occurring.

The rehabilitation of the ethos is as important as the rehabilitation of the individual. This is by no means an easy task where drinking is concerned. We go back to Nutt's (2012) argument in Chapter 1. The dominant attitude is that there is no problem with alcohol; rather, the problem lies with a few individuals who cannot 'handle' their drink, and we should not interfere with the general practice of drinking because of a few rogue individuals. The same attitude is prevalent in sport (of course, there are many exceptions, including some already mentioned in this chapter such as Arsène Wenger and Sven-Göran Eriksson). Such attitudes are untenable and fly in the face of the weight of evidence that an ethos that normalizes and celebrates alcohol use results in more problem drinking and more problem drinkers. If we want to reduce alcohol harms and alcohol problems in sport, we have to change the culture. Cairns et al. (2011) identified a number of typical aims in alcohol-reduction interventions, some of which were agent-centred, others of which were focused on what I have called ethos and others of which were a mix of both. These included 'strengthening of knowledge and skills to encourage healthy informed choices about alcohol', increasing awareness of 'risks and encouraging positive attitudes towards responsible alcohol consumption', a focus on the cultivation of 'social skills and cultivating resistance strategies against hazardous alcohol consumption' (for example 'building self-efficacy, training in higher order thinking and problem-solving') and the correction of 'misperceptions of alcohol norms such as peer dinking behaviours and prevalence of binge drinking' Cairns et al. (2011: 7). Importantly, they found that effective interventions must address both the individual and the environment in which the drinking occurs; in other words, the ethos. They argue that there should be specific focus on the social norms and peer alcohol use.

As mentioned earlier, an ethos or habitus is not static. The drinking culture in sport has changed over the years and is arguably less harmful than before (inasmuch as there is less routine heavy drinking that might interfere with fitness and performance). The growth of sport science in elite sport has served to curtail the opportunities to drink because athletes are monitored and tested on a daily basis. Any evidence of drinking alcohol or lack of sleep is picked up by the coaches and sanctions may follow. As such, athletes may choose only to drink alcohol at certain times, primarily when they are 'off duty'. This might exacerbate problems if athletes maximize their limited opportunities to 'party' and go 'over the top'. Another possible option is to seek other stimulants that might not register on any tests. Raheem Sterling, a young footballer, at the time with Liverpool FC, was photographed smoking a shisha pipe and inhaling what was thought to be nitrous oxide or 'hippy crack'. Neither is illegal, but both are condemned by the club nonetheless.[39] Moreover, at any given time the ethos is organic and changing, not least because of the clash between an intended ethos and an experienced ethos. Before concluding this chapter, I offer one final illustration of the confusing and inconsistent attitudes towards alcohol in sport. On 24 June 2010 the back pages of the *Daily Mirror*, a popular British tabloid newspaper, carried the headline 'Beer We Go'. The England football team had won their final qualifying group game at the 2010 World Cup in South Africa and the newspaper was in celebratory mood. After two inexplicably disappointing performances against the USA and then Algeria, during which time the team played way below the expectations and its brightest stars barely flickered, the media expressed a collective sigh of relief after the team improved enough to beat Slovenia by one goal and progress to the knock-out stages of the competition. In the next game England were beaten by their bitterest rivals, Germany, who despite fielding a relatively young and inexperienced side were more than a match for England's highly paid superstars. The backlash was ferocious. The media, ex-players, managers, pundits and commentators offered a range of different explanations for the abject failure of a team that went to the World Cup after a very successful qualifying campaign with high expectations. Explanations for the disappointment included systematic failures within the English game to produce technically gifted players, an excess of non-English players in the Premier League, player fatigue, a lack of passion and commitment connected to excessive salaries, and poor decision making by the manager, the Italian 'disciplinarian', Fabio Capello. Capello's role in England's poor performances was being questioned before their ultimate downfall at the tournament. Despite an exemplary record in qualifying for the tournament, problems emerged in the build up to the World Cup itself, and during the team's stay in South Africa. These included football issues involving squad selection, team selection, injured players and team formation. Capello's refusal to entertain a change in tactics, and his intransigence more broadly, became a target for criticism. He was accused of being stubborn, too strict and of heading a regime which produced demotivated and unenthusiastic players. His style, it was suggested, was unsuitable for the multi-millionaire footballers more used to self-indulgent lifestyles than the 'boot camp' atmosphere of the England training camp. The 'Beer We Go' headline, which hailed a short-lived renaissance for the England team, referred to a purported relaxation of Capello's 'no alcohol' rule for the players prior to the crucial third game against

Slovenia. That the players had their right to drink alcohol reinstated before this important match was widely reported as a media-led victory for common sense, and a triumph of British cultural habits evidenced by a demonstrable improvement in performance and results. Contrast this narrative with the press coverage of the England Rugby World Cup campaign in 2011 (mentioned above), where a relaxed attitude to alcohol consumption was considered to be a crucial factor in the failure of the team to perform well.

Summary

In this chapter I have argued that there is a pro-alcohol or perhaps 'pro-getting drunk' ethos in many sports. This ethos normalizes heavy drinking, particularly in relation to team bonding and celebrating. If we want to reform the risky drinking habits of individuals we have to reform the ethos of the practice community which encourages and celebrates such habits. This is by no means an easy task, but it is crucial if we are serious about reducing alcohol-related problems among athletes.

Notes

1 David Moyes, the then Manager of Manchester United FC, fined players for going out partying soon after an important loss for the team. http://www.manchesterevening-news.co.uk/sport/just-like-sir-alex-ferguson-6999090 (accessed 25/04/2014).
2 Under the influence. The damaging effect of alcohol marketing on young people. Report by the British Medical Association, September 2009. http://www.bma.org.uk/health_promotion_ethics/alcohol/undertheinfluence.jsp (accessed 25/04/2015).
3 http://www.mirror.co.uk/news/uk-news/paul-tobutt-inquest-groom-died-2029326 (accessed 19/05/2015).
4 http://www.telegraph.co.uk/education/educationnews/10889066/Teachers-in-a-drunken-brawl-on-school-trip-to-Barcelona.html (accessed 19/05/2015).
5 Halldorsson et al (2014: 311) found, with a large sample in Iceland, that 'adolescents that participate in formally organized sports clubs are less likely to use alcohol than those who do not'.
6 https://www.bostonglobe.com/opinion/editorials/2014/12/04/tries-new-tactic-fight-binge-drinking-transparency/SEoK8y45kKEkmAfedFNdOP/story.html (accessed 5/05/2015).
7 Kirby and Wintrup (2002: 50) discuss initiations and hazing (they provide a useful, but overlapping distinction between the two ideas), and argue that 'the concurrence of physical, mental and sexual abuse in such events places sport hazing solidly on the sexual harassment and abuse continuum proposed by Brackenridge (1997a)'.
8 http://www.bbc.co.uk/news/uk-england-gloucestershire-13795825 (accessed 25/04/2015).
9 Paul McGrath had a very successful professional football career while abusing alcohol, including playing while under the influence on many occasions.
10 http://www.dailymail.co.uk/sport/football/article-2522507/Arsenal-players-drunk-35-pints-won-double--Ray-Parlour.html (accessed 19/05/2015).
11 One of many incidents at the 2012 Olympic Games in London featured Belgian cyclist, Gijs van Hoecke, who was sent home from the Olympic Village after being photographed drunk and incapacitated by British tabloid press during a night out. The alcohol binge was a celebration or a 'blow out' after the pressure of taking part in the Games. http://www.independent.co.uk/sport/olympics/cycling/belgian-cyclist-gijs-van-hoecke-sent-

home-from-london-2012-olympics-after-drunken-pictures-appear-in-newspapers-8026407.html (accessed 7/11/2014).

12 http://www.telegraph.co.uk/sport/olympics/9399986/London-2012-What-goes-on-at-the-athletes-Olympic-village.html (accessed 13/08/2015).

13 http://www.walesonline.co.uk/news/wales-news/pub-door-staff-bar-henson-2124490 (accessed 8/07/2015).

14 http://www.theguardian.com/sport/2012/apr/01/gavin-henson-incident-plane-cardiff-blues (accessed 10/11/2014). http://www.theguardian.com/sport/2007/dec/05/rugbyunion.sport (accessed 12/11/2012).

15 http://news.bbc.co.uk/1/hi/wales/8516351.stm (accessed 18/02/2010).

16 https://www.facebook.com/pages/Andy-Powell-Appreciation-Society-For-Driving-A-Golf-Buggy-On-The-M4/301791227198 (accessed 5/4/2010).

17 He was commenting on the revelations that a prominent England rugby union player, Matt Stevens, had tested positive for cocaine. The force of the observation was that heavy drinking was fine, but drug taking was going too far. BBC Breakfast show broadcast 5 March 2009.

18 Mike Phillips, a key rugby union player for Wales, had been involved in a number of drink-related issues not long before the tournament and not too much time had passed since Andy Powell's golf buggy escapade.

19 http://www.bbc.co.uk/sport/0/rugby-union/15287034 (accessed 10/04/2013).

20 http://www.walesonline.co.uk/news/wales-news/drunk-rugby-players-called-disappointing-2046447 (accessed 19/05/2015).

21 http://www.bbc.co.uk/news/uk-england-somerset-23286282 (accessed 19/05/2015).

22 http://www.bbc.co.uk/sport/0/rugby-union/22290900 (accessed 7/11/2014).

23 http://www.bbc.co.uk/sport/0/rugby-union/24983640 (accessed 7/11/2012).

24 http://www.bbc.co.uk/sport/0/rugby-union/29305871 (accessed 12/05/2015).

25 See   http://www.independent.co.uk/sport/football/news-and-comment/footballers-we-know-what-you-did-this-summer-2307028.html,   http://www.theguardian.com/football/2012/aug/10/secret-footballer-undercover-premier-league (accessed 5/05/2015) and Anonymous (2012) for some examples.

26 Sheehan, P., 2009. Harry Redknapp wants his players to stay off the booze – win or lose. *The Sun*, http://www.thesun.co.uk/sol/homepage/sport/football/premteams/tottenham_hotspur/article2290512.ece (accessed 4/03/2009).

27 Moult, J., 2009. Don't you know who I am? *Mail Online*. http://www.dailymail.co.uk/news/article-1180014/Dont-know-I-England-Spurs-star-Ledley-Kings-jibe-arrested.html (accessed 11/05/2014).

28 So Peter Crouch, is this the right way to impress Fabio Capello and Harry Redknapp? *Mail Online*. http://www.dailymail.co.uk/sport/football/article-1221471/Peter-Crouch-risks-Harry-Redknapps-wrath-wild-night-town-Abbey-Clancy-Tottenham-team-mates.html (accessed 20/10/2014).

29 Stobart, G., 2009. Harry Redknapp on warpath after Spurs players' Dublin Christmas party. *The Telegraph*. http://www.telegraph.co.uk/sport/football/leagues/premierleague/tottenham/6841018/Harry-Redknapp-on-warpath-over-Spurs-players-Dublin-Christmas-party.html (accessed 12/02/2010).

30 http://www.mirror.co.uk/sport/football/news/qpr-booze-bender-dubai-players-1738275 (accessed 12/05/2015).

31 http://www.bbc.co.uk/news/uk-england-22545225 (accessed 19/05/2014).

32 http://www.bbc.co.uk/news/uk-england-23214468 (accessed 19/05/2014).

33 See Fuchs and Le Hénaff (2014) for a nuanced account of women's rugby and its ethos and attitudes to alcohol.

34 http://www.telegraph.co.uk/sport/cricket/international/australia/10116579/David-Warner-drank-Jagerbombs-and-vodka-before-punching-Joe-Root.html (accessed 19/05/2015).

35 See Krien (2013) for a disturbing insight into such issues in Australian professional sport.
36 http://www.independent.co.uk/news/uk/home-news/neknomination-craze-claims-fifth-victim-as-20yearold-bradley-eames-is-found-dead-after-downing-two-pints-of-gin-9131987.html (accessed 13/11/2012).
37 http://www.huffingtonpost.co.uk/2014/04/01/neknomination-rhiannon-scully_n_5067590.html?utm_hp_ref=uk (accessed 13/11/2012).
38 http://www.huffingtonpost.co.uk/2014/07/03/mamading-magaluf-video_n_5554565.html (accessed 12/05/2015).
39 http://www.independent.co.uk/sport/football/premier-league/raheem-sterling-laughing-gas-liverpool-will-not-punish-forward-over-hippy-crack-video-10176634.html (accessed 29/4/2015).

References

Adams, T., 1998. *Addicted.* London: Collins Willow.

Anderson, E., McCormack, M. and Lee, H., 2012. Male team sport hazing initiations in a culture of decreasing homohysteria. *Journal of Adolescent Research*, 27(4), 427–448.

Anonymous, 2012. *The secret footballer: lifting the lid on the beautiful game.* London: Guardian Books.

Bandura, A., 1971. *Social Learning Theory.* New York: General Learning Press.

Black, D., Lawson, J. and Fleishman, S., 1999. Excessive alcohol use by non-elite sportsmen. *Drug and Alcohol Review*, 18, 201–205.

Blum, L.A., 1994. *Moral perception and particularity.* Cambridge: Cambridge University Press.

Borsari, B. and Carey, K.B., 2001. Peer influences on college drinking: a review of the research. *Journal of Substance Abuse*, 13, 391–424.

Bourdieu, P., 1990. *The logic of practice.* Cambridge: Polity Press.

Brenner, J. and Swanik, K., 2007. High-risk drinking characteristics in collegiate athletes. *Journal of American College Health*, 56(3), 267–272.

Cairns, G., et al., 2011. Investigating the effectiveness of education in relation to alcohol: a systematic investigation of critical elements for optimum effectiveness of promising approaches and delivery methods in school and family linked alcohol education. Alcohol Research UK and University of Stirling Institute for Social Marketing/Open University. https://dspace.stir.ac.uk/bitstream/1893/11410/1/Cairns_2011_Investigating_the_Effectiveness_of_Education.pdf (accessed 8/09/2012).

Clayton, B., 2012. Initiate: constructing the 'reality' of male team sport initiation rituals. *International Review for the Sociology of Sport*, 48(2), 204–219.

Collins, T. and Vamplew, W., 2002. *Mud, sweat and beers: a cultural history of sport and alcohol.* Oxford: Berg.

Crundall, I., 2012. Alcohol management in community sports clubs: impact on viability and participation. *Health Promotion Journal of Australia*, 23(2), 97–100.

Davies, F.M. and Foxall, G.R., 2011. Involvement in sport and intention to consume alcohol: an exploratory study of UK adolescents. *Journal of Applied Social Psychology*, 41(9), 2284–2311.

Davis, P., 2012. The ladies of Besiktas: an example of moral and ideological ambiguity? *Sport, Ethics and Philosophy*, 6(1), 4–15.

De Visser, R.O. and Smith, J.A., 2007. Alcohol consumption and masculine identity among young men. *Psychology and Health*, 22(5), 595–614.

Denham, B.E., 2011. Alcohol and marijuana use among American high school seniors: empirical associations with competitive sports participation. *Sociology of Sport Journal*, 28, 362–379.

Diehl, K., et al., 2012. How healthy is the behaviour of young athletes? A systematic literature review and meta-analyses. *Journal of Sports Science and Medicine*, 11, 201–220.

Duff, C. and Munro, G., 2007. Preventing alcohol-related problems in community sports clubs: the good sports program. *Substance Use and Misuse*, 42, 1991–2001.

Dunning, E. and Waddington, I., 2003. Sport as a drug and drugs in sport. *International Review for the Sociology of Sport*, 38(3), 351–368.

Eccles, J.S. and Barber, B.L., 1999. Student Council, volunteering, basketball, or marching band: what kind of extracurricular involvement matters? *Journal of Adolescent Research*, 14(1), 10–43.

Edwards, L., Jones, C. and Weaving, C., 2013. Celebration on ice: double standards following the Canadian women's gold medal victory at the 2010 Winter Olympics. *Sport in Society*, 16(5), 682–698.

Flanagan, O., 1991. *Varieties of moral personality: ethics and psychological realism*. London: Harvard University Press.

Fleury, T., 2009. *Playing with fire*. Chicago IL: Triumph Books.

Ford, J.A., 2007. Alcohol use among college students: a comparison of athletes and non-athletes. *Substance Use and Misuse*, 42, 1367–1377.

Fuchs, J. and Le Hénaff, Y., 2014. Alcohol consumption among women rugby players in France: uses of the 'third half-time'. *International Review for the Sociology of Sport*, 49(3/4), 367–381.

Green, K., Nelson, T.F. and Hartmann, D., 2014. Binge drinking and sports participation in college: patterns among athletes and former athletes. *International Review for the Sociology of Sport*, 49(3/4), 417–434.

Halldorsson, V., Thorlindsson, T. and Sigfusdottir, I.D., 2014. Adolescent sport participation and alcohol use: the importance of sport organization and the wider social context. *International Review for the Sociology of Sport*, 49(3/4), 311–330.

Hamilton, J., 2008. *Beyond belief: finding the strength to come back*. New York: Faith Words.

Henson, G., 2005. *My Grand Slam year*. London: Harper Sport.

Kerr, Z.Y., De Freese, J.D. and Marshall, S.W., 2014. Current physical and mental health of former college athletes. *The Orthopaedic Journal of Sports Medicine*, 2(8), 1–9.

Kirby, S.L. and Wintrup, G., 2002. Running the gauntlet: an examination of initiation/hazing and sexual abuse in sport. *The Journal of Sexual Aggression*, 8(2), 49–68.

Martens, M.P., Watson II, J.C. and Beck, N.C., 2006. Sport-type differences in alcohol use among intercollegiate athletes. *Journal of Applied Sports Psychology*, 18, 136–150.

McDonald, B. and Sylvester, K., 2014. Learning to get drunk: the importance of drinking in Japanese university sports clubs. *International Review for the Sociology of Sport*, 49(3/4), 331–345.

McLaughlin, T., 2005. The educative importance of ethos. *British Journal of Educational Studies*, 53(3), 306–325.

Milgram, S., 1964. Group pressure and action against a person. *Journal of Abnormal and Social Psychology*, 69, 137–143.

Nutt, D., 2012. *Drugs without the hot air: minimising the harms of legal and illegal drugs*. Cambridge: UIT.

O'Brien, K.S., et al., 2008 Gender equality in university sportspeople's drinking. Drug and *Alcohol Review*, 27, 659–665.

Orford, J., et al., 2004. University student drinking: the role of motivational and social factors. *Drugs, Education, Prevention and Policy*, 11(5), 407–421.

Partington, S., et al., 2013. The relationship between membership of a university sports group and drinking behaviour among students at English Universities. *Addiction Research and Theory*, 21(4), 339–347.

Peck, S.C., Vida, M. and Eccles, J.S., 2008. Adolescent pathways to adulthood drinking: sport activity involvement is not necessarily risky or protective. *Addiction*, 103, 69–83.

Smith, K., 2012. *Kelly Smith: footballer; my story*. London: Bantam Press.

Sparkes, A., Partington, E. and Brown, D., 2007. Bodies as bearers of value: the transmission of jock culture via the 'Twelve Commandments'. *Sport Education and Society*, 12(3), 295–316.

Spijkerman, R., et al., 2007. The impact of peer and parental norms and behaviour on adolescent drinking: the role of drinking prototypes. *Psychology and Health*, 22(1), 7–29.

Sussman, S. and Arnett, J.J., 2014. Emerging adulthood: developmental period facilitative of the addictions. *Evaluation and the Health Professionals*, 37(2), 147–155.

Vamplew, W., 2005 Alcohol and the sportsperson: An anomalous alliance. *Sport in History*, 25(3), 390–411.

Wynn, S.R., et al., 1997. The mediating influence of refusal skills in preventing adolescent alcohol misuse. *Journal of School Health*, 67(9), 390–395.

Zhou J., O'Brien, K.S. and Heim, D., 2014. Alcohol consumption in sportspeople: the role of social cohesion, identity and happiness. *International Review for the Sociology of Sport*. 49(3/4), 278–293.

4 Role models and setting a good example

Introduction

In the last chapter, I argued that there was a problematic alcohol-tolerant or getting drunk ethos in many sports. Heavy drinking at certain times continues to be a practice in which even elite athletes participate, sometimes with, and sometimes without, the blessing of coaches, clubs and governing bodies. More often than not the drinking culture comes to our attention through the actions of one or two individuals who step out of line. Their actions are reported by the media (if the action and/or athlete are considered newsworthy), and depending on the nature of the behaviour they may be portrayed in a variety of ways. According to Lines (2001), sports stars are characteristically portrayed in the media as villains, fools or heroes, depending on the nature of their antics. Ray Rice's drunken attack on his fiancée in an elevator in Atlantic City in February, 2014, was given the full 'villain' treatment. Andrew Flintoff's drunken exploits, including his visit to Downing Street following the Ashes cricket victory in 2005 and the drunken trip on a pedalo in St Lucia in 2007, were portrayed as 'foolish', whereas Bradley Wiggins' celebrations mentioned in Chapter 2 were the well-deserved actions of a sporting hero. If, and when, there is moral condemnation of individuals, which may or may not be deserved, the language of 'role models' is often used. Athlete X is a role model and ought not to be setting such a bad example through his drinking or related behaviour. My aim in this chapter is to examine more carefully the use of the role model concept in moral evaluations of athletes in general, and of their alcohol-related behaviour in particular. I argue that we are entitled to expect reasonable standards of behaviour from athletes and that we are justified in condemning them when they fail to meet such standards. We are particularly justified in doing so in relation to excessive alcohol consumption, and the gamut of problems that often follow, because such behaviour has direct and indirect influence on others. We saw in the previous chapter that the example of high-status peers and drinking prototypes have been shown to influence the drinking of others.

Role models

In the last 7 years or so, since I became interested in the topic, there have been hundreds of examples of high-profile athletes falling foul of alcohol in one way or another in the UK alone. The USA, Canada and Australia provide further examples of individuals whose use of alcohol makes the headlines (sometimes repeatedly). When such individual athletes get into trouble for alcohol excess, or any other forms of deviant behaviour, it is largely, but not exclusively, *their* actions, personalities or character that are criticized and punished. The buck stops with the individual because they are the ones responsible for consuming the alcohol and engaging in any subsequent behaviour. I believe that the culture of drinking is protected by scapegoating these 'bad apples' in the way described by Nutt in Chapter 1. The moral opprobrium directed towards athletes who misbehave when drunk is often couched in the language of virtue and vice in general, and of role models in particular. High-profile elite athletes are described as role models because of their extraordinary feats of skill, endurance, speed and power, and their character in terms of determination, courage, perseverance and self-sacrifice. In some cases, perhaps increasingly rare, they are also applauded for exhibiting moral virtues such as fairness, loyalty, leadership and trustworthiness. A minority of very high-profile athletes may also be lauded as role models for representing a particular cause or charity.

Unfortunately, discussions about athletes as role models are generated as much, if not more, by athletes' bad behaviour; their vices rather than their virtues. Athletes who get drunk, take drugs or commit crimes are severely condemned by the media for setting a bad example. In the UK, the case of the professional football player Ched Evans has been played out in the media with a strong role model narrative. In the early hours of the morning after a night out drinking, Evans responded to a friend's (another professional football player) invite to join him in a hotel room because he had 'got a girl'. The intention was to have sex with the young woman who his friend had picked up on the night out. The woman accused both men of raping her and Ched Evans was found guilty and sentenced to prison for 5 years.[1] He was released from prison in October 2014 after serving half of his sentence. Media interest in his release from prison grew and focused specifically on whether he should be allowed to play football again. Initially, his club, Sheffield United FC, seemed willing to offer him a new contract, but as pressure mounted from sponsors, women's groups and various other constituencies who opposed his rehabilitation into professional football, the offer was withdrawn. The Professional Footballer's Association chief executive argued that Evans should be allowed to return to play because he had served his sentence.[2] The force of the opposition to Evans' return to football was that he was a bad role model. A convicted rapist ought not to be allowed to occupy the high-profile position of a professional footballer, or so was the view of many, including Nick Clegg, the then British Deputy Prime Minister. He said: 'when you take a footballer on, you are not taking just a footballer these days; you are also taking on a "role model"'.[3]

Despite their physical prowess and mental toughness, athletes are not immune from the frailties of body and mind which characterize the human condition. Loss of temper, aggression, cheating, violence, infidelity, selfishness, hubris, deceit, arrogance, immaturity, gluttony and lust, are all vices which visit athletes much like the rest of us. They are not saints! Given the pressures they are under, the conditions under which they operate, and so forth, it is perhaps to be expected that they often err. The difference is that for some athletes such failings are played out in the full glare of the media spotlight, and they face severe and perhaps unjustified criticism for failing in their responsibilities as role models. We, the viewing public, fans, media and academics, expect 'more' or 'better' from them. Given that the media has an appetite for scandal and that the behaviour of professional athletes is 'good copy', it is not surprising that negative narratives about the misbehaviour of athletes abound. The key issue is whether or not we are justified in giving athletes the status of role model in the first place and criticizing them when they let us down.

Virtue and character

When athletes are evaluated with respect to their role model credentials we use the familiar vocabulary of character, positive and negative, strengths and defects, or virtue and vice. If an athlete has behaved badly they may be described as undisciplined, selfish, dishonest, mean, cruel, immature, reckless, spiteful, lazy, argumentative, arrogant, violent, belligerent, deceitful or unprofessional, depending on the nature of the incident. As mentioned, athletes can also be kind, considerate, honest, caring, compassionate, courageous, brave, loyal, dedicated, faithful and trustworthy. Focusing primarily on the character of individuals in this way reflects a particular normative ethical approach to moral evaluation; namely, virtue ethics. Virtue ethics is an approach, or more precisely a set of approaches, to morality, which takes the character of the agent involved in moral action, their virtues and vices, as primary. In so doing, proponents attempt to articulate the grounds for praising virtuous characters and blaming bad ones. Virtue ethics is often contrasted with both deontology, which focuses on duties, and with utilitarian ethics, which focuses on the maximization of good consequences. It is an approach that is enjoying a renaissance in moral philosophy in general, and in sports ethics in particular.

Virtue ethics' genealogy is Aristotelian, but there are many contemporary versions. All, however, arguably share some ideas common to Aristotle's original account. Perhaps the most familiar features attributed to virtue ethics approaches is that they focus primarily on agents, on how one should be (being) rather than what one should do (doing). *Areteic* concepts – good, excellent and virtuous – are more prominent in virtue ethics than perhaps more familiar notions like rights, duties and obligations. According to McNamee (2008: 81):

> . . . an *areteic* conception of ethics focuses first and foremost on excellent character; on being a certain kind of person . . . . The right kind of person (i.e. a good one, a virtuous one) is one who does the right thing, for the right reason, at the right time, feeling the right way about it as they do it.

This distinction between the character of an agent and their actions is perhaps a little nebulous, but often features in the evaluation of athletes' behaviour. The distinction has recently been at the fore of racism-related incidents in the English Premier League. John Terry (English), captain of Chelsea FC, and Luis Suarez

(Uruguayan), then of Liverpool FC, were accused in separate incidents of making racist remarks to opponents during football matches. The Football Association of England found them both guilty of racism, of using racist language in an insulting way, but insisted that neither was a racist. They drew a clear distinction between the act and the character of the agent.[4] The distinction suggests that one may act in a certain way (e.g. racially abuse an opponent) but that such an action is not necessarily (but of course might very well be) a reflection of the type of person who committed the act, viz. their character. Certain situational or contextual factors may lead to a person acting uncharacteristically, a 'one off', but when a person repeatedly behaves badly we may conclude that there is a character flaw present (see discussion below). Such a distinction often crops up in relation to drunken behaviour, because alcohol distorts judgement and excessive consumption leads to behaviour that is 'out of character'.

Aristotle's account of character was set out in *The Nicomachean ethics* (2004) and represents a comprehensive account of the nature and scope of virtue. Aristotle talked about *aretē*, which has been translated to virtue, but encapsulated a broader range of excellences such as horsemanship, intelligence and moral virtues like courage. The complexity of Aristotle's account cannot be fully articulated here so only a rough sketch will be given. For Aristotle, virtues made sense in relation to some higher or further good. In other words, exercising virtue is to direct one's activities and character towards the achievement of some good or other. The *telos* (end) at which one directs one's virtues is *eudaimonia* or happiness. *Eudaimonia* was achieved, in part, by striving to live a virtuous life (a certain type of social/political life), and this striving involves cultivating and exemplifying good character. For Aristotle, the good life is not reducible to the narcissistic pursuit of pleasure. It is a matter of cultivating and exercising important virtues, like courage and justice, within a community. The virtuous person is praiseworthy and preferable to the bad *because* they exemplify and embody important dispositions like honesty, magnanimity and courage.

More recent accounts of virtue adapt and mould some of Aristotle's ideas to fit more comfortably with contemporary thought. For Pincoffs (1986), virtues, insomuch as they are manifest in a person's character, provide grounds for evaluation; that is, for preferring one person over another. Aristotle's conception of virtue shares this feature; that is to say, virtues provide grounds for evaluation; the just person is preferable to the unjust, the kind person preferable to the cruel, and the honest person preferable to the dishonest. The difference is that for Aristotle the preferences are predicated on the extent to which virtues contributed to and partly constituted a particular *telos*, namely *eudaimonia*. Pincoffs takes a broader perspective and argues that using virtues as the grounds for preferring one person over another need not be tied to an account of an overall *telos*. Pincoffs (1986: 7) uses the analogy of a ship; he suggests that for persons, like ships:

> . . . we do not need to know some supervenient common end before we can distinguish good from bad workings, so long as we understand the sorts of ends that will be pursued and the conditions under which they are to be pursued.

According to Pincoffs (1986: 7), therefore, the virtues are desirable not against some *telos*, but 'against a background of the common life, including the human tendencies that are aspects of that life'. Certain dispositions, such as justice, honesty and courage, are virtues in light of general facts about social life, such as communal living, family relationships, economic relationships and, of course, practices like sport. He suggests that virtues are understood as valuable in relation to the role or function they fulfil; for example, the virtues of a good father, compassion and care, differ from the virtues of a good soldier, courage, determination, obedience and cool-headedness. These virtues, insomuch as they are present, serve as grounds on which to evaluate the father and the soldier. We prefer brave soldiers rather than cowardly ones, and we prefer fathers to be gentle rather than cruel. Virtues, however, are not restricted to certain roles. They not only provide grounds for preferring persons in specific roles, but they provide the grounds for preferring certain persons and avoiding others at a more general level.

Another contemporary virtue theorist who features prominently in sports ethics literature is Alasdair MacIntyre (1985). For MacIntyre (1985), the virtues have a specific social role, primarily, but not exclusively, within social practices like sport. Similar to Aristotle, the virtues play a key role in accessing important goods, but for MacIntyre the goods in question are the 'internal goods' of the practice. The concepts of 'practice' and 'internal goods' have a very specific meaning for MacIntyre (1985: 187):

> By a 'practice' I am going to mean any coherent and complex form of socially established cooperative human activity through which goods internal to that form of activity are realized in the course of trying to achieve those standards of excellence which are appropriate to, and partly definitive of, that form of human activity, with the result that human powers to achieve excellence, and human conceptions of the ends and goods involved are systematically extended.

Sport is a paradigmatic example of the kinds of social practices where virtues are required to realize its internal goods (such as competitive intensity, skill and athletic excellence). For MacIntyre, three virtues are given particular prominence; namely, justice, courage and honesty. Exercising these virtues has important personal and social implications. It is only by playing sport virtuously that one realizes its internal goods. Exercising a virtue such as honesty also protects the integrity of the practice from the potential corrupting intrusion of external goods like money and fame, for example, refusing to cheat to secure financial rewards. Finally, the whole practice community is enriched by virtuous competitors and impoverished by bad ones. MacIntyre is perhaps unnecessarily reductive in his list of important virtues. There are a host of others which are important and laudable for citizens in general, and in relation to any specific role we might occupy, such as parent, teacher or athlete. According to Pincoffs (1986: 154): 'Reflections on the common life and its exigencies may yield conclusions about which virtues are especially to be encouraged and which vices are to be discouraged'. As such, he proposes a non-reductive and expansive list of virtues which include tolerance, benevolence, patience, fairness, integrity, kindness, love, compassion, cooperation, prudence, sensitivity, dignity, loyalty, magnanimity, persistence, determination and consideration. All are grounds for preferring one person over another, but are also important in the ways MacIntyre suggests above. Among the vices he identifies as destructive of human relations are deceptiveness, unfairness, callousness, insensitivity, the infliction of suffering and pain, injustice, lack of civility, cruelty and being weak-willed.

Using these insights from virtue theory we can begin to construct a case that athletes who exemplify certain virtues are preferable to those who exemplify vice, both in general and in relation to alcohol consumption and the problematic behaviour that often results from drunkenness. It would be better/preferable for the reasons sketched above if athletes exemplified virtue rather than vice. Many make the stronger claim that it would be preferable for athletes to exemplify virtue *because* they are role models. The force of this claim is that athletes have an additional obligation to be good because of their role, which gives them greater influence over others in the practice community of sport and beyond.

The role model's role

To be a role model is to play an important function in the personal social and moral development of other (often younger) individuals. From a virtue theory perspective, it is the growth of character in terms of the virtues mentioned above that is the crucial developmental goal. In order to explain the importance of role models in the cultivation and development of good character it is worth saying a little more about what virtues are and how they are acquired. Virtues are traits of character or qualities of persons, not of situations or actions. Flanagan (1991: 277) describes a trait as 'some sort of standing disposition to perceive and/or think and/or feel and/or behave in certain characteristic ways in certain situations'. In ascribing virtue, we are aiming to describe an element of a person's personality. As such, the virtues are dispositions or *tendencies* of a person to act in certain characteristic ways. The precise psychology of virtue is complex and contested. The stability and consistency of personality traits in particular was seriously threatened by experimental findings such as those of Stanley Milgram discussed in the previous chapter. Milgram (1964) was able to manipulate his subjects into behaving in unexpected (and vicious) ways which seemed to undermine our common-sense commitment to attributing behaviour to underlying character traits or dispositions. The results of these experiments and others, however, need not point to the absence of character traits, but tells us something very important about what such traits are actually like. Virtues are fundamental in moral agency, but they are not to be understood in a simplistic fashion. To describe someone as honest is not to suggest that they have some trait which at all times and in all circumstances produces honest action.

> Virtue theorists are right in thinking that moral responsiveness is mediated by a complex constellation of traits and dispositions . . . . But they are insufficiently aware of the degree to which the virtues and vices are interest-relative constructs with high degrees of situation sensitivity.
> (Flanagan 1991: 15)

Another important observation about the nature of the virtues is that the precise psychological antecedents of each virtue might be different. Compassion, for example, may be primarily an affective or emotional virtue, wisdom, primarily a cognitive or intellectual virtue, and industriousness, primarily a behavioural virtue. The implication is that when trying to cultivate virtues in children, or trying to change the habits of mature athletes, we need to understand the nature of the habit we are trying to develop (or get rid of). In other words, we need a picture of the kinds of characters we want – temperate, responsible and mature – and an insight into the psychology of such qualities, and perhaps more importantly their opposites (intemperate, irresponsible and immature).

So how do we become virtuous? For Aristotle (2004: 31), the virtues (including moral virtue) 'like crafts, are acquired by practice and habituation'. Virtuous character is not achieved through textbooks and lectures, but acquired through practice:

> It is the way that we behave in our dealings with other people that makes us just or unjust, and the way we behave in the face of danger, accustoming ourselves to be timid or confident, that makes us brave or cowardly.
> (Aristotle 2004: 32)

Flanagan (1996: 124) similarly argues for this practical, as opposed to theoretical, approach to the acquisition of moral knowledge; it is 'primarily a process of learning how: how to recognize a wide variety of complex situations and how to respond to them appropriately'. Cultivating good habits, among other things, involves seeking out the opportunity to practice them in various contexts and situations. As Aristotle (2004: 32) argues, 'we become just by performing just acts, temperate by performing temperate ones, brave by performing brave ones'. Most of the early moral training by parents is therefore aimed at fostering good rather than bad habits. Putman (1995) argues that children from a young age have the prerequisites of virtue, for example the capacity to empathize with others. Such empathy provides the foundation for a number of virtues like compassion, fairness and kindness. 'The parent's role is to fine-tune empathy both in terms of appropriate techniques and in terms of reinforcing the behaviour so it becomes a habit in the child's life' (Putman 1995: 178). For Aristotle, and other virtue theorists, the culture or community is vital in terms of providing the soil in which virtues (and vices) are cultivated. A good nourishing environment has a greater chance of producing good characters. In the last chapter I explained how important the ethos or habitus of sport was in cultivating drinking habits. An unhealthy alcohol ethos means unhealthy drinking habits.

Emulation and role models

Role models are crucial if virtues like honesty and kindness are to become an enduring disposition embedded in one's character. In order to become kind ourselves, we must see examples of kindness around us upon which we can base our efforts. In order for one to acquire virtue we should aim to practise in accordance with the example of a virtuous agent. Setting a good example, therefore, is particularly important for parents, teachers and coaches, and others, who seek to cultivate good habits among members of the family, school or sporting community. Sherman (1999: 37) argues that the 'force of a "role model" is that we learn through the concrete, through the narratives, stories and drama of someone who has been there, faced the music and made choices'.

The potential downside, of course, is that children may copy vice as much as virtues. This is the concern that lies behind the condemnation of athletes as bad role models. We do not want bad role models in the 'public eye' lest their presence serve to normalize or even legitimize bad behaviour. Luis Suarez, already mentioned in this chapter for his racism, also has a track record for biting opponents. After Suarez bit Chelsea's Branislav Ivanovic in 2013, the British Prime Minister David Cameron opined: 'I've got a seven-year-old son who loves watching football and when players behave like this it just sets the most appalling example to young people in this country'.[5] Inexplicably, Suarez repeated the offence at the World Cup in Brazil, in 2014, which suggests a character flaw. Bad behaviour, as well as good, can be copied. It is important therefore, that a message is given about which role models, or which traits or virtues in certain role models, deserve emulation, thus helping children and others recognize and identify worthy role models. Emulation is not simply duplicating or copying behaviour we see. It is a more complex process involving discernment and good judgement. According to Kristjánsson (2006: 44), emulation is itself a kind of virtue which involves striving for goods; that is:

> . . . goods that are morally worthy, or at least not morally unworthy. All in all, emulation turns out to be a complicated emotional virtue, the actualisation of which requires considerable acumen and moral discernment: the ability to feel, see and judge things correctly.

As with all virtues, emulation is acquired, and a key early role for parents and educators alike is to steer children away from morally 'unworthy' goods towards 'worthy' goods (see MacIntyre and Aristotle above). It is no easy task to help children discern the morally worthy from the unworthy in Western post-modern culture, but examples of good role models helps significantly. Celebrity or notoriety is a 'good' at which an increasing number of youngsters aim, and morality has little bearing on the means for its achievement. Individuals become rich and famous despite, or sometimes because of, behaving badly, and athletes like Suarez and others continue to enjoy the trappings of fame and wealth despite their antics. The disposition to copy, to envy and to covet must be steered in the direction of worthy 'objects'. This process involves individuals like teachers, parents and athletes (among others) exemplifying certain values and behaviours. The aim is that the ability or disposition to discern the worthy from the unworthy becomes instilled in children as a matter of good habit. Again the ethos of the community plays a crucial role in shaping and sustaining the behaviour and character of moral agents. If the prevailing ethos, moral atmosphere (Shields and Bredemeier 1995) or community (Kohlberg 1984) instantiates, celebrates and rewards virtue, individuals within that ethos are more likely to emulate, develop and sustain such virtues themselves. If the ethos celebrates drunkenness, misogyny, aggression and other vices, individuals within that ethos are more likely to emulate, develop and sustain such vices themselves. Developing a virtuous character, therefore, is not only good in itself, but acting and behaving well – exemplifying virtue – contributes positively to the ethos of the practice community and sets a good example to others.

Athletes as role models

When people talk of athletes as role models they may be making a number of different claims, some empirical (historical, sociological or psychological) and some normative (ethical). Until fairly recently, the cyclist Lance Armstrong, at least in some circles, was lauded as a paradigmatic example of a sporting role model. On the one hand, the assertion that he was a role model means that as a matter of fact Lance Armstrong had inspirational influence over a certain constituency of people who might include cyclists, cancer sufferers and others, who tried to 'be like him' in certain ways. Perhaps they strove to train harder, to bear misfortune with courage or to pursue goals despite setbacks. They might have tried to emulate his positive attitude, his great commitment to cycling, his charity work and his style (wearing Nike and/or Livestrong merchandise), among other things. In other words, what Lance Armstrong did influenced the attitudes, and even behaviour, of thousands if not millions of people. The particular size and scope of his influence might vary significantly from one individual to the next, of course, but it is possible, at least in theory, to discover some objective truth about the depth and breadth of his influence.

On the other hand, the claim that Lance Armstrong, or anyone else for that matter, is a role model, might entail a moral judgement, one that expresses a verdict about the quality of his character (or certain aspects of it). Role model is shorthand for some particular configuration of laudable qualities such as inspirational, courageous, dedicated, selfless, clean living, charitable and determined, or other worthwhile and admirable qualities of character. In this sense, to call someone a role model is to praise or prefer them (Pincoffs 1986). Sometimes, when used in this evaluative sense, role model might be prefixed by 'good' or 'bad'. A good role model is someone who exemplifies good qualities whereas a bad role model is someone who exemplifies bad ones. Unfortunately, as we know, Lance Armstrong became a bad role model overnight because it was discovered that dishonesty, deception and cheating were central to his story. He told lies, not white peripheral ones, but significant ones about the source of his sporting prowess.

Such qualities, cheating and lying, are *prima facie* unworthy and detrimental to sporting practices and it is preferable that others do not copy them.

The response of Jessica Ennis-Hill, Britain's Olympic gold medal winner in the heptathlon at the London 2012 games, to the Ched Evans case illustrates both the descriptive and normative elements of the role model concept. Ennis-Hill comes from Sheffield, and as a tribute to her achievements she had her name on a spectator stand at Sheffield United FC stadium. She asked that her name be removed from the stand if the club offered Ched Evans a new contract, commenting that:

> I believe being a role model to young people is a huge honour and those in positions of influence in communities should respect the role they play in young people's lives and set a good example. If Evans were to be re-signed by the club it would completely contradict these beliefs.[6]

She clearly believes that athletes do have influence *and* they ought to be worthy of emulation. There is little doubt that athletes are role models in a descriptive sense, but it does not necessarily follow that they should be role models in the normative sense.

Are we entitled to expect our athletes to be good role models?

Do athletes have a responsibility to be a role model? Is being an athlete a role that comes with additional responsibilities to be a role model? As we have seen, many think this is the case, but are they right? How might one construct an argument that athletes have such responsibilities? There are certain roles and professions, such as coaches, lawyers, politicians, teachers, doctors and the clergy, which are thought to be more demanding in terms of the character and conduct expected of those in the role. Such roles come with specific responsibilities or duties, not only to perform the actions that characterize the service, but also to exemplify personal and moral standards more broadly.

The claim that athletes (professional athletes in particular) have extended responsibilities for good conduct is not always articulated clearly, but there seem to be at least two types of argument that support it. First, there is the idea is that being a professional athlete is a role which carries some necessary duties to behave in a certain way. Arguments that focus on establishing duties in this way can be described as deontological. Being a professional athlete is similar to other professions and involves more than earning money for performing a role. There are additional moral standards to be upheld which extend beyond the execution of one's professional tasks (playing, teaching, prescribing and so forth). Although the argument that certain professions do indeed come with such extra duties (or perhaps these extra duties are definitive of a profession) has much to commend it, it is not easy to extend the argument to professional athletes. The profession shares little of the additional duty-generating features (such as dedicated and autonomous service to clients) of the traditional professions (Koehn 1994).[7] In sport the title 'professional' was originally used to distinguish between amateurs who played for 'the love of the game' and professionals who were paid to play. Of course, the adjective 'professional' has come to be used evaluatively to praise athletes, whether they are paid or not, for going about their endeavours in serious and committed ways. It is sometimes used, however, to describe an athlete who is willing to do whatever it takes to win, including 'bending the rules'.[8]

Such historical and semantic issues notwithstanding, professional athletes do have duties and responsibilities that extend beyond playing well. Whether they are definitive of, or a necessary aspect of, the role is a moot point, but sponsors, employers, clubs and governing bodies do make additional demands on athletes to make public appearances, talk to the media, represent their product or brand and engage in youth development work and community outreach projects and a whole range of other non-playing roles. Such expectations may be more or less explicitly articulated in contracts, agreements, codes of conduct and so forth. It is in reference to these 'extended' roles that drunken driving, sexual assault, domestic violence and other behaviours are incompatible. Certain behaviours may be explicitly forbidden by certain contracts or codes because they undermine the athlete's ability to portray the sport, the club, the nation and/or sponsor in a good light. The codes and contracts seek to formalize expectations in the form of duties. When in breach of these codes athletes bring the game/club/brand into disrepute. Sponsors are clearly committed to the idea that athletes can influence for the good and bad.[9] The golfers Tiger Woods and John Daly lost valuable endorsements because their respective behaviour was a potential threat to a brand image.

A second line of argument that athletes have extended responsibilities for good conduct has a distinct consequentialist tone. The additional responsibilities are generated in virtue of the potential influence occupiers of such a role can have on others, inside and outside the professional sport community. Their actions have the potential to cause harm. Consequentialists argue that we should all act in order to maximize good consequences and minimize bad ones. Athletes should therefore conduct themselves with this in mind.

Some disagree with the claim that athletes should be good role models. Mumford (2012: 99) agrees that athletes do have 'potential educative influence' and that this sphere of influence is greater than others not in the public eye, but this does not necessarily lead to any duty. If being in the public eye did carry such responsibilities it would attach to others such as rock stars and celebrities and would only attach to some athletes (the more prominent and well known) who as a *matter of fact* carry influence. Mumford (2012: 100) argues that there are no good reasons for obligating athletes to be role models. He claims, among other things, that: 'The status of "role model" is unreasonably conferred on to the athlete whether they want it or not' and: 'The role of "role model" is too demanding for anyone to fulfil'. I will discuss these two objections in order.

Athletes do not choose to be role models

There are at least two elements to this objection. The first consists of a straightforward rejection of duties we have not chosen. Athletes, who are often young and poorly educated, do not choose the burden of being role models; they want to play baseball or football, not play the role of moral exemplars. The issue is captured by contrasting quotes by the former professional basketball players Charles Barkley and Karl Malone respectively.

> I'm not a role model . . . . [T]he ability to run and dunk a basketball should not make you God Almighty. There are a million guys in jail who can play ball. Should they be 'role models? Of course not.
>
> Charles, you can deny being a role model all you want, but I don't think it's your decision to make. We don't choose to be 'role models', we are chosen. Our only choice is whether to be a good role model or a bad one. (Both quotes taken from Wellman 2003: 333)

Duties are not always matters of choice, as Malone indicates. In some cases, we are obliged despite our choices not because of them. Sandel (1984: 87) criticizes the idea of an 'unencumbered self', 'free to choose our purposes and ends unbound by . . . custom, or tradition or inherited status'. As mentioned above, it might be that certain duties come with a given role and are explicitly outlined in a code of conduct or contract (howsoever vaguely expressed). Others might be more indistinct or peripheral and come from the ethos, culture or community in which we live and work. We may be more or less aware of some of these until we are reminded of them when we or others transgress. Nevertheless, if there are such things as duties, they arise regardless of whether we have consented to them. For the duties to be meaningful, however, they must be justifiable. An athlete might object in the following way: 'I accept that being an athlete brings certain duties to execute my roles and responsibilities, but what I do in my private life is outside of this remit'. Some central responsibilities or duties are justified, but other peripheral ones are not. Whether an athlete is free to choose where they socialize, with whom, and for how long, whether they smoke, who they choose for sexual partners and what political affiliations they have, are all issues which have been brought to our attention by the press. Jack Wilshere, the young Arsenal FC player mentioned in Chapter 2, was photographed smoking while on holiday in Las Vegas in 2014. Although he broke no law, he apologized and made reference to his potential influence over others: 'I'm young and I'll learn from it. I realise the consequences it has and the effect on kids growing up'.[10] If an athlete is photographed at a club in the early hours of the morning or a campaign on social media objects to something they have done, then they may find themselves criticized for being bad role models and tried by the court of public opinion. Athletes cannot choose whether they have a duty to uphold certain standards of behaviour; however, they are entitled to have a fairly clear outline of the scope of these responsibilities. The cultivation of virtues like prudence will help athletes in the public eye avoid behaviours that are foreseeably contentious, like drinking excessively in nightclubs or driving under the influence of alcohol, using cannabis, smoking or inhaling laughing gas.

Expectations are too demanding

Mumford's (2012) second objection is that the burden of being a role model is too demanding for anyone, let alone athletes, to shoulder. According to Blum (1994: 158): 'What people regard as an "undue burden," however, and hence "what can be reasonably expected" is quite variable and can be deeply affected by their communities'. For Blum, the community is an identifiable group with a common moral outlook (or ethos), at least in relation to some particular feature such as charity or honesty. The ethos of a particular community reveals, to some degree, what is expected in terms of its members. In the case of professional athletes the intended ethos is demanding in terms of behaviour on and off the field. The experienced ethos does not sustain such high standards. The question remains whether these expectations are reasonable. According to Blum (1994), assessing the reasonableness of the demand is difficult because each community or ethos generates its own level of expectation and habits of behaviour.

Perhaps an illustrative example would help clarify. Consider two professional football clubs, X and Y. Club X has an ethos that demands a lot from its players in terms of conduct on and off the field. It encourages and cultivates an ethos of professionalism that includes exemplifying virtues such as honesty, trust and fairness. It discourages drinking and gambling and promotes certain positive values and expects players to be role models. Individuals are initiated into the ethos and are expected to conform to the demanding standards. Players who grow up in the club may find themselves complying with the standards and buying into the ethos. New recruits are expected to do the same, and if they are unwilling or unable to meet the demands they will be ejected regardless of their value as players. This club buys into Karl Malone's ideas about athletes as role models. Club Y has a very different approach. Its demands are fewer in scope and relate only to successful performance on the field. The criteria for continued membership of the club are largely based on competitive success, and other aspects of character and behaviour are not important unless they interfere with the main aim. The player's private lives are their own business and there are certainly no demands to be role models. This club's ethos is more like the attitude espoused by Charles Barkley. Each club clearly has a very different level of requirements in terms of the duties expected of players and staff: the former is very demanding, the latter less so. Which club has it right? This is a difficult question, but it is clear that *because* Club X's standards are more demanding it exemplifies greater virtue than club Y. Club X is more praiseworthy than Y because it expects robust moral standards from its players, and it would be preferable that Y followed suit regardless of whether the burden of doing so is more demanding. Good character is praiseworthy in part *because* it is demanding.

According to Aristotle (2004: 48), virtue:

> . . . to feel or act towards the right person to the right extent at the right time for the right reason in the right way – that is not easy, and it is not everyone that can do it. Hence to do these things well is rare, laudable and fine achievement.

Praise is rightly reserved for virtue and praiseworthy virtue is not easy. But how high should our expectations be? The issue here is about the level/consistency/standard of virtue we are entitled to expect from individuals in general, and our role models in particular. Aristotle's expectations for virtue seem particularly demanding for anyone, let alone young elite athletes. Mumford's (2012: 101) objection was that the role model idea entails very exacting if not impossible standards of goodness:

> The problem with 'role models' is their unreliability. A 'role model' is to be exemplary. They are to be emulated because they are completely or ideally good. But no one is likely to be able to live up to that ideal and when they do mess up in some way, we feel badly let down.

It is difficult to disagree with the second half of Mumford's claim; however, I am not convinced that we have to run with the articulation of role model offered in the first half. I wonder why we should set such high expectations on our role models? Of course, part of the idea of role model is that it exemplifies some (moral) worthwhile qualities, but it does not follow that these be so demanding that they are beyond the reach of most if not all moral agents (including, or perhaps especially, professional athletes).

The objection is grounded in concerns of psychological realism; that is, the putative responsibility to be a good role model is one that professional athletes (particularly the young) are ill-equipped (psychologically) to bear, and for that reason ought not to be obligated to standards way beyond their reach. Flanagan (1991: 32) argues that:

> ... when constructing a moral theory or projecting a moral ideal, make sure that the character, decision processing, and behaviour prescribed are possible, or are perceived to be possible for creatures like us.

We should not expect, he argues, that our practices and practitioners, in this case sports and athletes, are subjected to ideals that are simply unrealizable or impossible. Flanagan (1991: 26) argues that moral expectations 'which fail to meet certain standards of psychological realizability will fail to grip us, and in failing to grip us will fail to gain our attention, respect and effort'. We need not set our standards impossibly high, either in general or for athletes. We are not entitled to expect perfection, but asking them not to get drunk, drive under the influence, commit sexual offences and so on, seems perfectly reasonable. Being a role model is as much to do with exemplification of common standards of decency as with moral perfectionism. The exemplification and cultivation of the common virtues of decency is neither an unreasonable nor an unrealizable demand. Other admirable virtues that also contribute to a good ethos include prudence, responsibility, self-control and honesty. These are in addition to the sporting virtues of courage, loyalty, tenacity, perseverance, fairness and commitment that most elite athletes exemplify. Looking at common everyday virtues in this way can provide a robust, yet reasonable, framework for defending the position offered by Malone above.[11]

Blum (1994: 148–149) distinguishes between two uses of the term virtue. In one sense, virtue 'refers to a quality of character which is especially admirable' because it is above and beyond what is normally expected. Blum calls this type of virtue 'noteworthy' virtue. The second way virtue is used is to refer to more common or garden varieties that are to be expected of moral agents. These are, of course, morally good, but not particularly noteworthy, and may include such qualities as honesty and decency (although it seems to me their absence or opposites are noteworthy). Blum (1994: 149) calls this type 'ordinary' virtue. Classifying virtues in this way relates to their particular instantiation. It's not that there are some 'ordinary' and some 'noteworthy' virtues, although some, like courage, are more likely to be noteworthy. There are ordinary and noteworthy acts of honesty, compassion and generosity. The particularities of the case tell us which label is best suited. Blum (1994: 149) argues that: 'In general, I would suggest that every virtue has both noteworthy and ordinary manifestations, depending on the circumstances'. Take the virtue of generosity. To be generous is always beyond what might be deemed as one's duty. Some acts of generosity are particularly noteworthy, others less so. Nevertheless, ordinary virtues are important and praiseworthy. Virtues, as has been mentioned, are acquired through a complex process that includes habituation, teaching, practise, emulation and exemplification. A good role model might only exemplify ordinary virtue, but this is praiseworthy and important. Athletes who exemplify the ordinary virtues of common decency and prudence are crucial to our practices. They can be role models and help shape a morally decent ethos.

Ordinary and noteworthy sporting role models

I have argued that we are entitled to expect a certain level of ordinary virtue from our athletes and we should encourage and celebrate noteworthy virtue. It is certainly not difficult to provide an account of athletes exemplifying ordinary, but important, virtues. Treating people with respect, courtesy and politeness in dealings with other members of the team or club, including coaches, fellow athletes and ancillary staff, are important ordinary virtues which are nevertheless commendable and contribute to an overall positive ethos. Being punctual, cooperative and reliable are all qualities worth emulating. So too are dedicating oneself to the pursuit of excellence in sport through the application of one's talent, determination and dedication; and demonstrating loyalty to a team and to battle against fatigue in order to succeed. Building a long and successful career in sport, performing regularly to a high standard and securing the associated intrinsic and extrinsic goods; to respect the best traditions of one's club and country, and to respect one's family and community by not bringing themselves and the sport into disrepute are all important qualities of role models. These are by no means excessively demanding yet incredibly praiseworthy.

In 2011, during the Rugby World Cup, Wales' young captain Sam Warburton was heralded as a role model for a number of reasons, including his responsible attitude to alcohol and his role in cultivating a similar attitude throughout the team.[12] Having a responsible attitude to alcohol consumption, having the courage to withstand temptation and the strength of character and confidence to resist certain pressures to engage in negative behaviour, such as initiations and drinking rituals, are praiseworthy and even noteworthy in sport. Andy Murray's abstinence appears to be noteworthy, certainly in the British press's eyes. Conversely, the absence of vices like impatience, intolerance, rudeness, arrogance, gluttony and greed is preferred to their presence, and athletes can be good examples in this regard too. Desisting from the numerous problematic drink-related behaviours, ranging from stealing golf carts, getting hit by buses, attacking wives and girl-friends, violence, criminal damage, lewd behaviour to sexual impropriety and infidelity, are all reasonable expectations. Modelling habits that instantiate respect for one's own well-being by not consuming more alcohol (or any other unhealthy behaviour) than is deemed wise by the medical profession is also important.

There are many ways in which athletes can exemplify noteworthy virtue and be good role models too. There are countless examples of sporting excellence which become part of sporting folklore (as do extraordinary examples of vice). Examples of athletes who exhibit courage in the face of significant challenges on and off the field abound. Their perseverance and stoicism in light of overwhelming odds does them credit and their narratives provide a rich source of material for moral lessons. Professional sportsmen and women can also exhibit moral excellence by rejecting vices like corruption, cheating, deception, bad sportspersonship, vio-lence and other blights on the professional game despite overwhelming pressures. Recent revelations about suspected doping in athletics suggest that clean athletes are particularly commendable in rejecting dubious performance enhancing meth-ods. Refusing to engage in premeditated acts of cheating and deception, often in opposition to a corrupt ethos, are noteworthy. To make a stand against racism, homophobia and sexism also exemplifies noteworthy virtue.

There are other ways in which the narratives of athletes can inspire and set an example of noteworthy virtue. The famous actions of John Carlos and Tommie Smith at the 1968 Olympic Games showed courage, solidarity and a commitment to important values like freedom and equality. These African-American athletes stood on the medal podium and raised a black gloved fist in the air in protest about the treatment of black people in the USA at the time. In the current context, I would like to offer some other, perhaps less likely, candidates as role models. Athletes like Tony Adams (1998), Sugar Ray Leonard (2011), Theo Fleury (2009) and Josh Hamilton (2008) are all overcoming problems with alcohol and drugs. Adams' pub-lic admission of alcoholism, his determination and courage to seek help, and his commitment to helping others through his Sporting Chance clinic, is a story well worth telling (Adams 1998). Role models like Adams are particularly worthwhile, and provide a counterpoint to the glorified or sensationalized stories of individuals like George Best. Other athletes, for example Andy Murray, who choose abstinence where alcohol is concerned are noteworthy role models in relation to alcohol.

It seems to me that if we do not set the bar excessively high we are entitled to expect athletes to behave well and exhibit good character in terms of ordinary virtue. When they do this they are being good role models. This helps to create a community or ethos which exemplifies ordinary virtue. If they do not we are entitled to criticize them and describe them as bad role models. Athletes can also exemplify noteworthy virtue, and when they do they are candidates for being excellent role models.

Summary

When individual athletes get drunk and behave badly they are criticized, often using the role model narrative. I have argued that it is reasonable to criticize athletes in this way. In so doing I have advanced a particular conception of role models that does not place too heavy a burden on professional athletes, or anyone else for that matter. A role model is someone who exemplifies virtue, even ordinary virtue. Exemplifying ordinary virtue is important because people who are decent and honest are preferable (Pincoffs 1986) to those who are not. Moreover, society in general and sporting communities in particular depend on ordinary virtue, and role models play a crucial role in the development of such virtues in others. Athletes are in a position of greater influence than many others, and they should recognize the implications of the greater consequence their behaviour might have and act accordingly. Exemplifying good conduct where alcohol is concerned is part and parcel of being a role model.

Notes

1 http://www.bbc.co.uk/news/uk-wales-17781842 (accessed 26/11/2014).
2 http://www.theguardian.com/commentisfree/2014/oct/15/ched-evans-sentence-rape (accessed 18/12/2015).
3 http://www.bbc.co.uk/sport/0/football/29656157 (accessed 26/11/2014).
4 See Jones and Fleming (2007) for an extended discussion of the difference in relation to racism in sport.
5 http://www.telegraph.co.uk/news/politics/david-cameron/10020060/David-Cameron-Luis-Suarez-was-appalling-role-model-for-my-son.html (accessed 28/11/2014).
6 http://www.theguardian.com/sport/2014/nov/13/jessica-ennis-hill-name-stand-ched-evans-contract-sheffield-united (accessed 28/11/2014).
7 See McNamee (2011) for a synopsis of Koehn's (1994) account of what constitutes a profession.
8 For a discussion about the use of amateurism and professionalism as moral language for evaluating sport, see Morgan (1993).
9 Woods lost deals with Gatorade and AT&T, among others, after his admission of infidelity in 2010. http://news.bbc.co.uk/1/hi/business/8540167.stm (accessed 10/12/2014). Daly was dropped by Wilson and Reebok while in rehab in 1997 (Daly 2007: 154).
10 http://www.telegraph.co.uk/sport/football/teams/arsenal/10993547/Arsenals-Jack-Wilshere-sorry-for-smoking-on-holiday-after-the-World-Cup.html (accessed 12/12/2014).
11 Wellman (2003) uses the ingenious and very effective heuristic of an imaginary dialogue between these two athletes to argue for the conclusion that there is a duty to be a good role model qua person, but there are additional special responsibilities which come with the privileged position. In the imagined voice of Malone he argues that 'What this means is merely that you should recognize that along with the privilege of your exalted standing comes a special responsibility to be mindful of your actions and the heightened influence they have on others' (Wellman 2003: 336).
12 http://www.bbc.co.uk/sport/0/rugby-union/15135951 (accessed 18/12/2014).

References

Adams, T., 1998. *Addicted.* London: Collins Willow.

Aristotle., 2004. *The Nicomachean ethics.* Trans. J.A.K. Thomson. London: Penguin.

Blum, L.A., 1994. *Moral perception and particularity.* Cambridge: Cambridge University Press.

Daly, J., 2006. *My life in and out of the rough.* London: Harper Sport.

Flanagan, O., 1991. *Varieties of moral personality: ethics and psychological realism.* London: Harvard University Press.

Flanagan, O., 1996. *Self expressions: mind, moral and the meaning of life.* Oxford: Oxford University Press.

Fleury, T., 2009. *Playing with fire.* Chicago. IL: Triumph Books.

Hamilton, J., 2008. *Beyond belief.* New York: Faith Words.

Jones, C. and Fleming, S., 2007. 'I'd rather wear a turban than a rose': the (in)appropriateness of terrace chanting amongst sport spectators. *Race, Ethnicity and Education,* 10(4), 401–414.

Koehn, D., 1994. *The ground of professional ethics.* London: Routledge.

Kohlberg, L., 1984. *Essays on moral development. Volume 2. The psychology of moral development.* San Francisco: Harper and Row.

Kristjánsson, K., 2006. Emulation and the use of role models in moral education. *Journal of Moral Education,* 35(1), 37–49.

Leonard, S.R., 2011. *The big fight: my autobiography.* London: Ebury Press.

Lines, G., 2001. Villains, fools or heroes? Sports stars as 'role models' for young people. *Leisure Studies,* 20, 285–303.

MacIntyre, A., 1985. *After virtue.* London: Duckworth.

McNamee, M., 2008. *Sports, virtues and vices.* London: Routledge.

McNamee, M., 2011. Celebrating trust: virtues and rules in the ethical conduct of sports coaches. In: A. Hardman and C. Jones, eds. *The ethics of sports coaching.* London: Routledge, 23–41.

Milgram, S., 1964. Group pressure and action against a person. *Journal of Abnormal and Social Psychology,* 69, 137–143.

Morgan, W., 1993. Amateurism and professionalism as moral languages: in search of a moral image of sport. *Quest,* 45(4), 470–493.

Mumford, S., 2012. *Watching sport: aesthetics, ethics and emotion.* London: Routledge.

Pincoffs, E.L., 1986. *Quandaries and virtues: against reductivism in ethics.* Kansas: Kansas University Press.

Putman, D., 1995. The primacy of virtue in children's moral development. *Journal of Moral Education,* 24(2), 175–183.

Sandel, M., 1984. The procedural republic and the unencumbered self. *Political Theory,* 12(1), 81–96.

Sherman, N., 1999. Character development and Aristotelian virtue. In: D. Carr and J. Steutel, eds. *Virtue ethics and moral education.* London: Routledge, 35–49.

Shields, D.L.L. and Bredemeier, B.J.L., 1995. *Character development and physical activity.* Champaign, IL: Human Kinetics.

Wellman, C., 2003. Do celebrated athletes have special responsibilities to be good role models? An imagined dialogue between Charles Barkley and Karl Malone. In: J. Boxill, ed. *Sports ethics: an anthology.* Oxford: Blackwell, 333–336.

5   Drinking too much and punishment

Introduction

In Chapter 3 I argued that many athletes (professional and amateur) engage in patterns of drinking which should concern us, and that many sporting cultures have an ethos that condones and encourages excessive drinking, especially on certain occasions. This does not mean that 'anything goes'; because sporting authorities will punish athletes for drink-related behaviour if they feel they have overstepped the mark. There are countless examples of athletes who have been punished for their behaviour when drunk. For example, the Welsh rugby union player, Andy Powell, arrested by the police for stealing a golf cart, was subsequently punished by the Welsh Rugby Union. His crime came at the end of an organized post-match celebration involving heavy drinking.[1] Similarly, Andrew Flintoff, the England cricketer who got into difficulties on a pedalo in the West Indies in 2007, was fined for his drinking behaviour along with five other players.[2] My aim in this chapter is to examine the practice of punishing athletes for drink-related behaviour. First, I will examine the concept of punishment and its various justifications. Second, I examine some of the philosophical and ethical issues associated with punishing someone who is drunk, particularly in light of a culture that promotes getting drunk. Finally, I argue that the most important decision in drink-related offending is often the decision to start drinking. As such, the widespread and collective intention to get drunk embedded in the ethos of many sports should be a key focus for reform.

The concept of punishment

Fundamentally, punishment is an action or a practice that involves the deliberate infliction of suffering of some kind on another human being. Given that the infliction of suffering is normally to be avoided and the actions and character of those who inflict such suffering are condemned, the concept of punishment requires explanation and its use requires justification. According to Honderich (1989), anything described as punishment must involve suffering or some such thing (other candidates may include discomfort or the deprivation of some good, and in sport may include fines, suspensions or termination of contract). More than this, the suffering has deliberately and intentionally been brought about. As such, punishment shares characteristics similar to other morally dubious acts such as revenge, assault, abuse or cruelty. Punishment, however, is legitimate, and its legitimacy is partly to do with the authority of the punisher and partly to do with certain important and definitive characteristics of the recipient. Punishment is partly legitimized because it is carried out by someone who has the *rightful* authority to inflict suffering. Without such authority, common 'punishment' acts such as fines, incarceration or archaic practices like beatings are simply theft, assault, violence, cruelty or kidnap. The other legitimizing condition of punishment, according to Honderich (1989), is that the recipient is an offender; that is, someone who has committed an offence and *deserves* to be punished. Punishment can be summarized thus:

> . . . an authority's infliction of a penalty, something involving deprivation or distress, on an offender, someone who has freely and responsibly broken the law or rule, for that offence. (Honderich 1989: 9)

This account provides us with a thumbnail definition of punishment, but not yet a justification for its use in general, or in any given instance in particular. We may ask further questions. What purpose does it serve? What are the authorities hoping to achieve by punishing? In relation to sport, what are the authorities hoping to achieve by fining, dropping or banning athletes for alcohol-related offending?

According to Honderich (1989) there are three standard types of justification for punishment; punishment as retribution, punishment as a deterrent and punishment to rehabilitate. The first is backward-looking and justifies punishment as a form of retribution for the act committed by the offender. Punishment as retribution implies that the punishment is 'deserved by offenders for what they willingly did' (Honderich 1989: 6). 'Deserved' is meant in two ways: first, that they were guilty, they actually committed the offence, and, secondly, the type or amount of punishment meted out stands in proportionate relation to the offence. So an athlete who broke a curfew and had a few drinks committed an offence and deserves punishment, but might not deserve a lifetime ban. The 'eye for an eye' maxim implies that retribution ought to involve the infliction of similar or equivalent suffering on the offender as the offender visited on his or her victim(s). Of course, most systems of punishment avoid this direct formula but maintain that the punishment should fit the crime. If the punishment is too lenient we feel that justice has not been served.

The second type of justification for punishment is forward-looking and is closely associated with the utilitarian moral theory proposed by philosophers such as Jeremy Bentham and John Stuart Mill. Utilitarians believe an action is right if it contributes to a greater balance of pleasure over pain, or satisfaction over dissatisfaction, or good over evil. Punishment serves a utilitarian goal by deterring or preventing future bad actions (offending). It does so in two ways. First, punishment *deters* by identifying to potential offenders the likely consequences of their bad actions. As such, it makes potential offenders self-interestedly reflect on their intentions and motives and choose a course of action that will avoid the unpleasant consequences of punishment. If a person has murder on their mind, the threat of life imprisonment or the death penalty should deter them from such actions. Punishment needs to be sufficiently unpleasant if it is to work as a deterrent. Secondly, punishment *prevents* offending by rendering a particular offender incapable of further offending through incarceration or expulsion. While suspended, an athlete cannot reoffend, provided it was an on-field offence (for example, Mike Tyson's boxing license was revoked for biting his opponent's ear; therefore, he was not able to repeat the offence while banned).

The third standard approach to the justification of punishment also focuses on the reduction of offending. The assumption here is that offending can be reduced, not simply by rendering the offender incapable of further offence, but by changing or reforming the offender's character in some way. It is a 'kind of cure' for wrongdoing (Aristotle 1980: 32). After being punished the offender is less likely to reoffend because they have been reformed, rehabilitated or learnt their lesson. Rehabilitation of offenders has both inherent and instrumental value. Punishment rehabilitates the offender by improving their character and making them a better person, but in so doing there is a further payoff because once rehabilitated there will not be any further offences (at least not by them). Honderich (1989) argues that in most cases at least two types of justification are used in conjunction with each other. For example, the deterrent and rehabilitation accounts might be used to justify a suspension of an athlete who has offended. While suspended the offender will be unable to commit further offences and will be minded to rethink their future conduct (rehabilitated). Luis Suarez has now been suspended three times for biting an opponent, with each offence drawing increasingly more severe punishment. Whether punishment is effective, or any particular type more effective than another (severity versus leniency), is of course a matter of heated debate. The high reoffending rates of people leaving prison and the examples in sport of repeat offending, such as Suarez on the field, and athletes like Danny Cipriani and Gavin Henson off the field, call into question how effective punishment is in either preventing or rehabilitating (at least for some people).

What is the offence?

One of the key questions connected to punishing athletes for offences related to alcohol is what exactly counts as an offence. An offence is generally thought to mean a wrongful act and punishment is meted out when someone is judged to have committed such an act. Alcohol-related offences in sport come in various guises and manifest themselves in relation to some framework or other. In sport there are at least four possibilities. First, there are regulative and ancillary rules and codes within sport that inform athletes about acceptable and unacceptable behaviour. In terms of what athletes are allowed to ingest, there is a long list of substances proscribed by the World Anti-Doping Agency. In some sports, mainly motorsports, alcohol is forbidden for obvious safety reasons, but most sports do not forbid alcohol, and having a 'sip' of brandy or whisky before a game or at half-time was (and at certain levels may still be) common. It remains a tradition to sip champagne during the final stage of the Tour de France. It is not unheard of, but rare, for alcohol offences to occur in relation to these rules. Secondly, athletes are governed by other rules and regulations mentioned in the previous chapter, such as codes of professional conduct and contractual obligations to employers including sponsors, clubs, governing bodies and so on. These may all have clauses relating to acceptable and unacceptable alcohol consumption and other behaviours. When athletes represent their country at the Olympic Games, for example, they may be governed by regulations that apply to them while 'on duty' for their country. These rules may also make reference to the particular laws of the land. Thirdly, establishments and institutions such as hotels, training venues and athlete villages (at the Olympic Games) may have certain rules about behaviour and conduct in general, and about alcohol in particular. Finally, the law of the land specifies a whole range of behaviours that constitute offending in relation to alcohol, including drunk and disorderly conduct, being drunk and incapable, driving under the influence of alcohol, underage drinking and, perhaps, laws about where and when alcohol can be consumed. Offending in light of these latter laws is usually a matter for the police and criminal justice system, but sporting authorities might take additional action against an athlete arrested for being drunk and disorderly because their behaviour is construed as a breach of contract or is thought to bring the game into disrepute.

Some of the expectations concerning drinking are clear and instantiated in formal codes, rules or laws with accompanying information about what sanctions might be incurred if breached. An individual might be ignorant of a particular law or rule, but they are bound by it nonetheless. Other expectations might not be so clearly demarcated in rules or laws because it is impossible to spell them all out. As McFee (2004: 107) argues, no rule or law can deal with 'every situation unequivocally' because there is no '*all*, no finite totality of possible cases'. It is unlikely that it is stipulated anywhere that 'one ought not to operate a pedalo while drunk' as happened to Andrew Flintoff, or 'one ought not to get hit by a bus while drunk', as happened to the rugby union player Danny Cipriani, yet athletes can expect to be punished if such events happen as a result of their drinking, particularly if the incident gets into the public domain. In such cases an appeal might be made to the 'spirit' of a general principle of good behaviour. The principle itself might be loosely outlined in contracts and codes, and couched in language such as 'bringing the game into disrepute' or '(un)professional conduct'. Such open-ended caveats allow authorities to exercise judgement and discretion with respect to decisions regarding punishing athletes' behaviour in general, and with respect to alcohol in particular.

Alcohol and offending among athletes

The most high-profile incidents, those which make it into our newspapers and onto our television screens, usually with a 'bad role model' narrative, tend to involve not only the excessive consumption of alcohol, but public drunkenness and/or additional bad behaviour. In this respect alcohol differs from substances like cocaine, ecstasy or marijuana. In many countries consumption (possession) of such drugs is criminalized. Even ex-athletes are subjected to the public's, or perhaps more accurately, the media's chagrin if they have used drugs.[3] Neither excessive alcohol consumption nor severe intoxication is necessarily a criminal offence. In the UK, being drunk is only an offence if an individual is deemed incapable, or is behaving in a disorderly manner, or is engaged in other prohibited behaviour such as driving while drunk.

I have argued that the intention to get drunk is part of the experienced ethos in sport, sometimes facilitated by coaches (celebration/team bonding), and by sponsors supplying free alcohol. There is a significant degree of leniency and tolerance of drunkenness at certain times, and the range of behaviours that often accompany drunkenness, such as uncharacteristic bluntness, unguarded comments, tactlessness and inappropriate flirtation. Sometimes the ethos demands that the whole team turn a collective 'blind eye' to alcohol-fuelled bad behaviour, an attitude sometimes encapsulated in the old adage 'what goes on tour, stays on tour'. In some cases the behaviour might only be deemed as 'offending' if the media publicize it; that is, when private behaviour is made public. Given the proliferation of phone cameras, closed-circuit television and the appetite for compromising photographs of misbehaving athletes, this is happening increasingly. The media exposure and publicity will play a significant role, not only in drawing attention to the incident but perhaps in 'creating' the offence. This is what happened in the example discussed in Chapter 3 with the England rugby team. During the Rugby World Cup in New Zealand in 2011, members of the England team, including its captain, were photographed at a nightclub drinking and participating in the entertainment provided.[4] As I mentioned, Martin Johnson, the England team coach, refused to take any action because he had given the players permission to go out and did not feel any breach of discipline had occurred; in other words, there was no offence. The Rugby Football Union (RFU) took a different view and subsequently punished Tindall. The Rugby Players' Association objected to the harsh punishment, arguing that no offence had been committed; he had complied with the curfew. The RFU disagreed and Rob Andrew (RFU operations director) justified the punishment: 'Tindall's actions reached a level of misconduct that was unacceptable in a senior England player and amounted to a very serious breach of the EPS [Elite Player Squad] Code of Conduct'.[5] The court of public (or media) opinion is neither a reliable nor a fair way of deciding whether an offence has occurred and whether punishment should follow.

This case further illustrates two important issues. The first is that there is a clear difference between the alcohol ethos that the governing body intends, and the one embodied in the player's behaviour. From the player's perspective getting drunk and participating in puerile bar-room entertainment was fine as long as they met the curfew. The governing body saw things differently. The second issue relates to the reach of any code of conduct. The fact that Mike Tindall already had two convictions for driving under the influence of alcohol did not trouble the RFU, in terms of either selecting him or making him the team captain. Those offences were deemed to be irrelevant to his role and not a matter for the RFU. In the UK an athlete's employer or national governing don't seem particularly concerned with a player's drink driving convictions. In 2005, Jermaine Pennant, an English footballer with Birmingham City FC, was convicted of driving under the influence of alcohol. At the time, he was banned from driving for previous offences and was therefore given a custodial prison sentence as punishment. After a short time in prison he was released, but had to wear an electronic tag. He continued to represent his club and played with the tag.[6] The behaviour did not, however, incur further censure under the guise of 'unprofessional conduct' or 'bringing the sport/club/country into disrepute'. A conviction for drink driving does not constitute an offence as far as some sporting authorities are concerned, at least in the UK, but being photographed in a nightclub drinking often does. Stuart Lancaster, the former England rugby union coach, took alcohol-related incidents more seriously. He dropped Danny Care from the England squad for the 2012 Six Nations Championship after he pleaded guilty to drink driving. He has also excluded Manu Tuilagi from the 2015 World Cup squad after he was convicted of an early morning assault on a taxi driver and two female police officers.[7]

Sponsors might also be more concerned with the potential damage to their brand of having a convicted drink driver endorsing their products. John Daly, the American golfer, was dropped by his sponsors, Wilson and Reebok, while in the Betty Ford Center because of his problems with alcohol (Daly 2006). Whether a criminal offence comes to be judged as an offence in the eyes of sporting authorities and merits further punishment seems to depend on a number of mitigating and aggravating factors. As mentioned, sporting authorities might not take any further action against a player who has been convicted of driving under the influence. Luke McCormick killed two young children while driving under the influence of alcohol, and is now back playing professional football in the UK after serving part of a 7 year custodial sentence, and Lee Hughes is also back playing professional football after serving a custodial sentence for causing death by dangerous driving.[8] The picture is mixed, and different in different sports and in different countries. An athlete may find themselves punished for a relatively minor offence – for example, being out late or being photographed being out late – but have no action taken against them by their employers for a drink driving conviction.

Alcohol and moral responsibility

As mentioned, being drunk is not an offence, or at least not one that is likely to come to light unless further offences are committed, such as missing curfew, being hungover at training and so on. Getting drunk inevitably increases the chances of further offending (as discussed in Chapter 1). Because alcohol can have such a significant effect on one's personality, its consumption, along with that of other mind-altering substances, raises crucial questions with regards to offending and punishment. Recall how Honderich (1989) argues that for punishment to be justified the person who commits the offence must be an offender. In other words, they must deserve the punishment. The drunken or hungover athlete deserves punishment for being late to training, performing badly, damaging property, stealing or causing injury or death by driving under the influence. Moreover, the threat of punishment should deter the drinker from offending. From a philosophical perspective the matter is more complex. I will discuss the issue of desert first, before returning to the effectiveness of punishment as a deterrent in alcohol-related offending.

> The culpability of an offender in his offence, we may say, depends on two things: the harm caused by his action and the extent to which he can be regarded as having been free and responsible in his action. (Honderich 1989: 31)

The first part of the claim focuses on at the consequences of the action; what was the harm? In the foregoing we have seen that the putative harm caused by drinking athletes varies significantly, from minor reputational harm or breaches in team discipline, to significant physical harms through violent conduct and in some cases death by driving under the influence. In this part of the chapter, however, I am more interested in the second element of Honderich's claim. It raises complex legal, psychological and philosophical questions about free will and responsibility in general, but also in relation to offences committed under the influence of intoxicating substances like alcohol and other drugs in particular. The presence and effects of mind-altering substances on individuals raises important and emotive questions about whether offenders under the influence of such substances are 'in control' of their actions and thereby responsible for them. Alcohol changes the personality, which is of course part of the reason we drink it, but it has detrimental effects on motor skills and decision-making abilities long before we feel its effects.[9] If drinking continues, reaction time suffers, and we lose more control over our behaviour. It is these effects that often lead people to do things they would not have done otherwise. Some (perhaps most) of the incidents mentioned throughout this book involve athletes doing something they would not have done when sober. Because alcohol can significantly affect behaviour, in some cases being drunk *is* offered *and* accepted as grounds for different treatment or mitigation. Most people who have been drunk have pleaded with spouses or friends for forgiveness for misdemeanours committed when drunk. More significantly, in some criminal cases the presence of alcohol might be a crucial factor in the way decisions are made. A victim, but not the perpetrator, in a rape case, may be judged incapable of acting voluntarily (of giving consent) because of drink.

Does this change have any moral significance in terms of responsibility for actions when drunk? We have already noted that a drunken person might be deemed incapable of consenting. Moral responsibility is the property that makes agents justifiable targets for praise or blame and, more specifically in the current context, punishment. Moral responsibility indicates whether individuals deserve certain treatment or not. For Aristotle, moral responsibility applies to actions which are not compelled nor done in ignorance; that is, actions which are knowingly and freely chosen.

As we have seen, the consumption of alcohol in general, and being drunk in particular, can compromise free choice and voluntary action. Being drunk undermines one's ability in many aspects, including making rational judgements and being 'suitably sensitive to situation-sensitive moral concerns' (Vargas 2005: 269). In other words, the presence of alcohol inhibits the faculty of reason, impedes moral conscience, undermines the capacity for informed decision making and has a clear causal role in the kind of offending discussed above. By their own testimony, people who offend when drunk claim that they were 'not in control', 'did not know what I was doing', 'things got out of hand' or 'I didn't mean to do it'. Ray Rice's fiancée stressed they were 'drunk and tired' at the time of the heavily publicized assault by the NFL star, and said she could not remember much about the incident.[10] In Aristotelian terms, alcohol impedes and undermines both freedom and knowledge, which are central planks of voluntary, and thereby responsible, action. Often these problems can be exacerbated by features of the context, as we saw in Chapter 3. Alcohol, combined with peer pressure, a heavy drinking ethos, an important victory and underlying aspects of one's own character, can propel an individual into behaving in a way they would not normally behave.

Does any of this this amount to an excuse? Not necessarily, because even if we accept an offender is ignorant of the consequences of their behaviour, Aristotle argues that we may hold the offender responsible for their ignorance. In relation to a drunken offence, Aristotle (2004: 62) is clear, alcohol-induced ignorance is their fault '. . . because the source of the action lay in the agent himself: he was capable of not getting drunk, and his drunkenness was the cause of his ignorance'. If, when drunk, the individual misjudges their ability to drive or miscalculates how much they have had to drink, such ignorance is their own fault and ought not to count in mitigation. Current thinking mirrors ancient thought in this respect. Morse (2011: 181) argues that 'the law is generally unforgiving if a defendant lacked a required mental state as a result of voluntarily getting drunk'. Even if we accept that at a specific moment in time an intoxicated person acts involuntarily, we nevertheless intuitively believe that person made bad choices leading up to the particular incident and was responsible for those decisions. Vargas (2005: 269) describes this as 'tracing':

> Tracing is the idea that responsibility for some outcome need not be anchored in the agent or agent's action at the moment immediately prior to outcome, but rather at some suitable time prior to the moment of deliberation or action.

In this respect, we might accept that at the specific time alcohol did have a detrimental effect on the autonomy of the individual, but at some point we believe they were in a position to make a rational and informed decision. Luke McCormick's (the footballer who killed two young children while driving under the influence of alcohol) actions are anchored in 'his earlier decision to drink in circumstances where he might feel the temptation to drive while drunk' (Vargas 2005: 270). In other words, we believe that previous to driving while under the influence of alcohol there was a point at which the offender could have made a decision not to drink, or to ensure that there was no risk of driving while still under the influence of alcohol.

Tracing back through a series of events to some previous decisive point, therefore, seems intuitively sensible. There are, however, a number of difficulties both in general and especially in particular cases (Vargas 2005). The example of the rugby union player Andy Powell, who drove a golf cart down the highway in the early hours of the morning, effectively illustrates a number of difficulties. If we accept that he was very drunk at the time he returned to the hotel, and this significantly undermined his ability to make rational choices, we can reasonably ask two questions about his actions. First, was it reasonable to expect him to foresee that these *specific* consequences might occur if he were to get drunk? After all, as far as we know he had not done such a thing before. This is a crucial factor with alcohol consumption. Given the nature of the substance, it might be very difficult to predict its specific effects; that is, beyond making you drunk. One might reasonably foresee that drinking too much will get you drunk, but not that it will lead you to specific types of problematic behaviour such as infidelity, violence or theft. Morse (2011: 182) argues that:

> It is clear, however, that many people who create grave risk to others without awareness of that risk when drunk were not aware when they became drunk that they would be in this situation while drunk.

If we believe that he ought to have been aware of the risk of such consequences, or at least some similar reckless behaviour, as a result of drinking, we might ask a second question: at which precise point in the evening was it reasonable for him to have foreseen such consequences? At which point in time, as he got more intoxicated, was he able to act differently? This is by no means a straightforward issue, yet a fundamentally important one. The problem relates not only to the intoxicating effects of alcohol, but also to the cumulative and progressive impairment of autonomy. Can we be sure, either conceptually or empirically, at which point an individual fails both the knowledge and freedom conditions because of intoxication? The boundaries are vague between competence and incompetence, but what is certain is that the drinker is not a good judge of his own competency. A particularly tiresome characteristic of a drunk is their insistence that they are not drunk despite overwhelming evidence to the contrary.

There are two issues here, one more important than the other. The first is a theoretical point about whether we can identify (trace) the decisive point prior to the offence, when the offender was still capable of making rational decisions, and after which they were, due to drink, incapable of acting rationally. Identifying such a point is important in order to establish culpability, although precision is impossible in practice. Drunk or drunkenness is a concept like *tall* or *heap* that philosophers describe as vague. They are vague because it is not clear at which precise point a person becomes tall or, as in the sorites paradox, at which point a few grains of sand become a heap. We might agree on obvious cases of drunkenness but find difficulty agreeing at which precise point a sober person turns into a drunken one. Getting drunk is an incremental process which starts with the decision to take a drink of alcohol, but depending on the individual's constitution each subsequent sip of alcohol has an effect. Most drinkers identify the turning point in terms of drinks; for example, 'it was the third drink' or 'the whiskey chaser' that tipped the balance. The important fact, however, is not when an individual subjectively feels they became drunk, but the point at which alcohol rendered them incapable of rational decision making and voluntary action. Pinpointing the precise moment that competence becomes incompetence, or responsibility becomes irresponsibility, is difficult, both subjectively (individuals rarely recognize that point themselves) and objectively. Nevertheless, the judgement has significant implications for drink-related offending because someone (often a jury) has to decide whether a person was incapacitated in some way by alcohol.

   This leads me to the second issue. The reality is that those in authority required to make a judgement are not likely to attempt such a fine-grained analysis. They have to make a judgement in light of the evidence in front of them. In some offences there are objective measures of when alcohol constitutes impairment. In the UK, police breathalyse suspected drivers, and if a certain threshold is met the driver will be arrested. Until recently this was 35 micrograms of alcohol per 100 millilitres of breath, but Scotland has decided to lower the threshold to 22 micrograms in line with most European countries.[11] The measure reflects a level at which it is thought the ability to drive safely is compromised. Lowering the limit reflects a more cautious approach and that, if driving, people should not drink at all and certainly should not try to drink 'up to' the limit.[12] In most other cases a judgement about how drunk or impaired an offender is draws on different evidence. This might include how many drinks they had, how long they had been drinking and their observable behaviour (for example, being unsteady or slurring their words). The authorities are unlikely to be concerned about which precise point in the incremental process of getting drunk the offender was capable of taking, and ought to have taken, a different decision; that is, either not to engage in, or to have drunk to levels that increased the risk of, offending behaviour.[13]

Is setting out to get drunk morally problematic?

If getting drunk carries such risks, why is the decision to get 'hammered', 'smashed', 'pissed', 'off my face', 'wasted', 'leathered' or 'mangled' still so popular and acceptable, particularly in comparison to the decision to take a line of cocaine or an ecstasy tablet?[14] Notwithstanding the legal issues, our attitudes towards alcohol are significantly different to those towards other drugs that may have similar effects. The morally salient or significant decision where drugs are concerned is the decision to consume them; they provoke a 'moral panic' in comparison with alcohol. With alcohol we only become concerned if something further happens as a result of consumption. A tragic incident involving a young athlete illustrates this difference. In June 2012, a promising young British cricketer, Tom Maynard, died after being hit by a train near Wimbledon Park tube station in London, at 5 am. His car was stopped by police and he fled on foot over the railway lines, the implication being that he did not want his breath to be tested. Pathology reports showed that he was nearly four times over the drink drive limit for alcohol, but the findings that dominated the story was that he had also taken cocaine and ecstasy, and that he may have been a regular cocaine user for over 3 months prior to the incident. The amount of alcohol consumed was largely ignored as the drug-taking became the main focus. The journalist and ex-cricketer, Steve James, commented in his newspaper column:

> Maynard had been drinking, but worse still for the grieving family, a post-mortem examination revealed that he had taken cocaine and ecstasy, and hair samples indicated he might have been a 'habitual' user in the three months before his death.[15]

It is not clear, at least not in terms of their causal role in his death, why drugs are 'worse still'. His consumption of alcohol was significant, arguably decisive, in his death, given the amount he drank and that he died trying to evade the police who would likely breathalyse him. The ethos of heavy drinking among cricketers, and the routine consumption of high levels of alcohol on a night out by young British adults, largely escaped scrutiny. It was the spectre of a possible drug culture that dominated the headlines, with some inside the game denying that drugs were a problem and others calling for tougher drug-testing regimes. Alcohol got off relatively lightly as it always does despite its role in the countless deaths of young people (see Chapter 1). Maynard had been disciplined by his employer, Surrey County Cricket Club, a week before because he had been run over and injured himself while drunk during a night out.[16] In the case of drugs, the expectation is that one should never take them again, whereas with alcohol the expectation is that one should behave better next time, or take it easy. The decision to drink, or at least the decision to drink so heavily, however, is as important as, or more significant than, the decision to take drugs, and may even have been a contributory factor in the drug taking. When drunk, taking drugs might seem like a good idea and the resources to resist are depleted by alcohol. Recently, Jake Livermore, a player for Hull City FC (an English Premier League club at the time), tested positive for cocaine. His manager, Steve Bruce, commented:

> We're all let down, from everybody concerned with the club, and everybody concerned with football. We're all let down. But the biggest one, he's let down is a blossoming career. He's let himself down. Being tarnished with that is awful and he'll have to live with the consequences of that.[17]

The player was banned by the Football Association and may face a charge of gross misconduct and be sacked by his club. The reaction, and perhaps the formal proceedings relating to the incident is, as usual, disproportionate in comparison to that surrounding offences committed by footballers when alcohol is involved.

If we accept alcohol's causal role in bad behaviour and that autonomy, reason and rational decision making are slowly undermined from the first sip of alcohol (and are significantly undermined with larger quantities), the decision to drink is a significant one. The habit of making severe intoxication the aim of a night out, as is custom and practice in sport, is perhaps *the* morally significant choice. Such a decision carries foreseeable and unforeseeable risks. The decision to drink too much (although legal) seems wholly irrational given the associated negative consequences, particularly for individuals like Tom Maynard, Danny Cipriani, Gavin Henson, Ray Rice and many others inside and outside of sport. To paraphrase Flanagan (2011: 273), excessive drinking can defeat the prospects of '*eudaimonia*, to flourish, to find meaning and fulfilment', yet the behaviour as I have argued throughout this book is common, tolerated and, in some contexts – including sport – encouraged and celebrated. Behaving badly when drunk might be condemned and punished, but punishment loses some of its potential power in the face of alcohol. Once drunk, athletes (or anyone else) lose the capacity to reason appropriately and punishment as a deterrent is weakened. Furthermore, even if one is severely punished for an offence, the punishment might be targeted at the behaviour (violence or some such) not the intoxication. Even if one is punished for being drunk and disorderly, the hope is that the offender will not repeat the 'disorderly' behaviour rather than the 'drunken' behaviour.

There is considerable reluctance to acknowledge that the culture of getting drunk is problematic. It is easier to scapegoat the one who gets into trouble rather than reflect on the general and often collective choice to get drunk. There may be many reasons for this. One reason is that it is a popular choice embedded in Western culture and in the ethos of many sports. Drinking to excess is a tradition, pastime and hobby for many and people want to protect their right to get drunk ('it's my right and as long as I don't harm anyone' and so on and so forth). Another reason is the belief that the decision to get drunk is not foundational in the way I suggest above. Even when drunk, each action is one for which the agent *is* fully responsible. The offending action *is* a result of choice; the agent *could* have done otherwise but chose not to and is culpable for decisions made howsoever drunk. In other words, getting extremely drunk does not necessarily lead to 'offending' because not everyone offends when drunk. It is the character of offenders not alcohol that is to blame. Offenders are *offenders* in the true sense of the word because despite being drunk they knowingly and willingly offend. 'Only bad characters or those who can't hold their drink offend when drunk, the rest of us are fine!' Although it is true that not everyone who gets extremely drunk commits offences, a significant number of offences, particularly certain kinds, are committed by people who have been drinking. Drinking inevitably increases the risks and we cannot confidently predict what we may or may not do when drunk because, as mentioned, we cannot predict what set of circumstances might arise. The prudent approach is to reduce the risk of offending and victimization by not getting drunk. For some this may mean avoiding alcohol altogether.

Back to punishment

The punishment meted out to athletes for drink-related offending might be aimed at restoring justice, deterring further offending (either by the offender or others by way of example) or reforming or rehabilitating the character of the offender in some way, or a combination of these. We have seen that for punishment to be justified the offender must be responsible for the offence inasmuch as they knew what they were doing and could have done otherwise. Intoxication makes this judgement difficult, but being drunk is not accepted as an excuse for diminished responsibility, at least for the offender. If it is true that alcohol undermines our ability to make rational decisions, any intervention (punishment) aimed at behavioural change must look to target the rational agent before they are adversely affected by drink. No one, when sober, would envisage that they need the threat of punishment to abstain from urinating on a train, stealing a golf cart, attacking their fiancée or some such. Furthermore, when drunk the threat of punishment is diminished. It is only when someone can muster their rational capacities, weigh up the consequences of their actions, evaluate risks and so forth that they can decide that running in front of a bus, drinking on an aeroplane at 7 am or evading police are all bad decisions. The sensible goal, therefore, is to target the decision to get drunk and look to stop individuals from embarking on a course of action that might lead to bad decisions which, at worst, may cost them or others their lives. There is evidence that an increasing number of elite athletes are making the decision to abstain from alcohol and a number of governing bodies, coaches and clubs are seeking to cultivate an (intended) ethos where getting drunk is no longer acceptable. A change in the culture is crucial and will mean a reduction in alcohol-related problems in sport. A cultural change, however, will not mean that no athletes will get into trouble again. There are some individuals who will ignore any rules or threats and continue to drink regardless. I discuss such individuals in the next chapter.

Summary

In this chapter I have made the case that the decision to drink in general, and the decision to get drunk in particular, has significant implications. Alcohol undermines our capacities to make sensible decisions and it is the bad decisions that usually constitute the offences for which athletes are punished. Had they not been drunk, the likelihood is that they would not have committed those acts. The prudent thing to do would be not to drink so much, or, perhaps for some, not to drink at all (I pick up this idea in the next chapter). Punishing athletes for their behaviour when drunk might be ineffective for the reasons I have mentioned. They may not have any intention to offend, but by drinking heavily they significantly increase the risk of getting into trouble (victims or perpetrators) they did not seek or foresee. I argued in Chapter 3 for a reform of the ethos and in Chapter 4 for individuals to take more responsibility for their drinking. In the next chapter I look more closely at certain individuals who seem to have a pattern of problems and examine how they are dealt with in various sporting contexts.

Notes

1 http://news.bbc.co.uk/1/hi/8515002.stm (accessed 13/01/2015).
2 http://news.bbc.co.uk/sport1/hi/cricket/england/6464251.stm (accessed 13/01/2015).
3 http://news.bbc.co.uk/sport1/hi/tennis/8329193.stm (accessed 13/05/2014).
4 http://www.theguardian.com/sport/blog/2011/sep/15/dwarf-throwing-england-rugby (accessed 29/01/2015).
5 http://www.telegraph.co.uk/sport/rugbyunion/international/england/8883289/Mike-Tindalls-England-career-is-over-after-25k-fine-for-serious-misconduct-at-Rugby-World-Cup.html (accessed 6/01/2015).
6 http://news.bbc.co.uk/1/hi/england/london/4396747.stm (accessed 8/1/2015).
7 http://www.telegraph.co.uk/sport/rugbyunion/international/england/11608554/Manu-Tuilagi-to-miss-World-Cup-after-assaulting-police-officer.html (accessed 28/05/2015).
8 http://www.theguardian.com/football/2014/nov/12/footballs-sacking-offences-drugs-dangerous-driving-rape-ched-evans (accessed 8/1/2015).
9 http://pubs.niaaa.nih.gov/publications/RethinkHoliday/NIAAA_NYE_Fact_Sheet.htm (accessed 30/01/2015).
10 http://www.washingtonpost.com/blogs/early-lead/wp/2014/11/28/after-ray-rices-reinstatement-janay-rice-speaks-out-about-elevator-incident/ (accessed 30/01/2015).
11 http://www.bbc.co.uk/news/uk-scotland-30329743 (accessed 30/1/2015).
12 It seems that the new tougher limits in Scotland are having a significant impact on the economy. It seems bar sales have dropped by 60%. The industry is of course concerned about its profits, but the figures illustrate that most people are applying the letter of the law, rather than its spirit, in terms of alcohol's role in impeding driving ability. http://www.independent.co.uk/news/uk/home-news/scotlands-new-drinkdriving-law-is-so-successful-its-damaging-the-economy-according-to-bank-of-scotland-report-10173764.html (accessed 30/04/2015).
13 The Association of British Travel Agents has launched a campaign to educate young UK travellers about the dangers of falling from hotel balconies while on holiday. A growing number of young UK citizens on vacation in popular resorts in Spain, Turkey and Greece are being seriously injured or killed falling (or jumping) from hotel balconies, and the UK Foreign Office believes that alcohol plays a central role in these accidents. Given that the *raison d'être* for taking a vacation at such resorts for young people is often the heavy drinking and partying (resorts are marketed as party venues), one wonders whether a campaign should be aimed at reducing drinking or being more careful when drunk. http://www.telegraph.co.uk/travel/travelnews/9476958/Warning-over-hotel-balcony-falls.html (accessed 24/08/12).
14 Wiktionary lists well over 100 terms and expressions to describe getting drunk. http://en.wiktionary.org/wiki/Appendix:Glossary_of_drinking_slang (accessed 23/01/2015).
15 http://www.telegraph.co.uk/sport/cricket/counties/9904264/Cricket-prodigy-Tom-Maynards-father-says-after-inquest-His-lifes-worth-remembering-for-more-than-these-drug-findings.html (accessed 9/1/2015).
16 http://www.bbc.co.uk/news/uk-england-london-21588586 (accessed 9/1/2015).
17 http://www.telegraph.co.uk/sport/football/teams/hull-city/11610449/Steve-Bruce-Telling-Jake-Livermore-hed-failed-drugs-test-was-hardest-conversation-Ive-had-with-a-footballer.html (accessed 28/05/2015).

References

Aristotle, 1980. *The Nicomachean ethics.* Trans. W.D. Ross. Updated J.L. Ackrill and J.O. Urmsom. Oxford: Oxford University Press.
Aristotle, 2004. *The Nicomachean ethics.* Trans. A.K. Thomson. London: Penguin.
Daly, J., 2006. *My life in and out of the rough.* London: Harper Sport.

Flanagan, O., 2011. What is it like to be an addict? In: J. Poland and G. Graham, eds. *Addiction and responsibility*. Cambridge: MA: MIT Press, 269–292.

Honderich, T., 1989. *Punishment: the supposed justifications revisited*. London: Pluto Press.

McFee, G., 2004. *Sport, rules and values: philosophical investigations into the nature of sport*. London: Routledge.

Morse, S.J., 2011. Addiction and criminal responsibility. In: J. Poland and G. Graham, eds. *Addiction and responsibility*. Cambridge: MA: MIT Press, 159–199.

Vargas, M., 2005. The trouble with tracing. *Midwest Studies in Philosophy*, XXIX, 269–291.

6 Alcohol misuse, abuse and disorder

Introduction

Throughout this book I have focused largely on social factors that contribute and create an ethos or *habitus* which normalizes the excessive consumption of alcohol. Although I have argued that the social context or ethos can push or entice people to develop problematic drinking habits and behaviours, a person's drinking habits must surely depend on their choice; perhaps not always a rational one, but their choice nonetheless. Problem drinkers could change, and many do, if a strong enough reason presents itself. There are certain individuals in sport, like in all areas of life, however, who seem to have particular difficulties with alcohol. They come to our attention because they are serial offenders in terms of behaving badly when drunk, or show other symptoms of dependency in terms of the amount and frequency of use. They have developed, or perhaps are at risk of developing, a dependency on alcohol which threatens their career, well-being and ultimately their life. Perhaps the best footballer of all time, the career and subsequent life of Diego Maradona was, and remains, plagued by alcohol and other drug problems. The UK footballers George Best, Paul Gascoigne, Tony Adams and Paul McGrath, the Canadian ice hockey player Theo Fleury, the boxer Sugar Ray Leonard, the basketball player Vin Baker and the Australian rugby union player Kurtley Beale are just a few of the other familiar high-profile athletes who are (or were) self-confessed alcoholics or have had well-documented difficulties with alcohol. Such individuals are particularly perplexing because their actions are self-defeating and irrational, particularly given what they have to lose (or did lose) as a result of excessive drinking. Why are they not able to resist the desire to drink and prioritize their careers, families and well-being? Why are some athletes not deterred or rehabilitated by the system of punishment? What should be done about them? These questions are the main focus of this chapter.

We are perplexed by the behaviour of individuals like those mentioned above because we think they should have more self-control. They should be able to resist their desires. According to Frankfurt (1971), the ability to resist or to choose which of our desires to act upon is a unique feature of human beings. In fact, it is this ability to care about which desires we act upon or the ability to form 'second-order desires' that separates us from other species (Frankfurt 1971: 6). Human beings are uniquely capable of wanting their wants, preferences, desires, tastes and appetites to be different than they are. We are able to reflect on our first-order desires and form second-order desires. For example, we may have two conflicting desires: the desire for another cold beer and a desire to drink sensibly. When we reflect on these desires we may conclude that it is the latter desire that we want to act upon and therefore choose to abstain. We are generally able to turn one desire into 'our will' and act on it (Frankfurt 1971). Despite our second-order desires to want to behave in a certain way, sometimes we may not be able to override one of our first-order desires. Such a failure is often described as a weakness of will. Frankfurt discusses the example of an addict who, despite not wanting to be addicted to a drug, and despite identifying strongly with the first-order desire to refrain rather than the desire to use, remains unable to abstain. In such a case, Frankfurt (1971: 13) argues, it seems plausible to say that the addict is being moved by a force 'other than his own, and that it is not of his own free will, but rather against it . . .'. In other words, it is not that the addict's will is weak; it's not his will at all. Over the years, addicts' irrational behaviour has increasingly, at least in some circles, come to be thought of as a compulsion beyond their control. It is a result or symptom of a condition or an illness that causes them to use, regardless of their reflective desire not to.

Personality disorder

Irrational behaviour is fairly common; for example, many of us are prone to eating more than is good for us. We do not worry too much about this even though the long-term consequences might be serious. For some, like the athletes mentioned above, their irrationality seems beyond the 'normal' or 'acceptable' boundaries, and cause them significant problems. The desire for the drink (or drug, sex or gambling) at certain times overpowers all other concerns and considerations, and even if they have a second-order desire to abstain it is ineffective. Consequently, the consumption results in significant problems that can be described as the symptoms of addiction. Matthews (2007: 1) argues that: 'It is not rational, for instance, knowingly to act against one's own long term self-interest, or to pursue minimal benefit at a great risk or great cost'. When individuals' wills seem pathologically irrational and exceed normal bounds of irrationality, medical or health-led wisdom concludes that they have a 'clinical problem'. They are described as having a personality disorder (PD) or, more specifically, a substance abuse disorder or addiction (Matthews 2007: 2). According to Pickard (2011a), a PD occurs when one's behaviour deviates markedly from the norm. One's personality is the characteristic way in which 'we are inclined to think, feel, and act in response to particular circumstances, as well as more generally' (Pickard 2011a: 181). We all have a personality and have aspects of it that we might prefer not to have; for example, not to be so shy, or so quick to anger, and so on. A disordered personality, however, occurs when:

> . . . a set of characteristics or traits that make a person the kind of person they are causes severe psychological distress and impairment in social,

occupational, or other important contexts: the ways a person is inclined to think, feel, and act do them harm, directly or via the effects they have on relationships, work and life more generally conceived. Diagnosis of a PD requires that these characteristics or traits be long-standing, pervasive, difficult to control or change, and markedly different from cultural expectations. (Pickard 2011a: 181)

According to Pickard, PD is at the extreme end of a continuum of normal personality. It is the extremity of the characteristic rather than the characteristic *per se* that signifies disorder. We all have sexual desires, but in the case of Mike Tyson and Sugar Ray Leonard, they talk of excessive or compulsive desires which led to extreme sexual behaviour that put them at risk of consequences ranging from unwanted pregnancy, marriage break up and life-threatening sexually transmitted diseases like HIV.[1] There are many types of PD clustered into three categories colloquially known as the 'mad' (cluster A: paranoid, schizoid and schizotypal), the 'bad' (cluster B: narcissistic, borderline, histrionic and anti-social) and the 'sad' (cluster C: obsessive compulsive, avoidant and dependent) (Pickard 2011a: 182). Those who have problems with alcohol, and other substances and behaviours, might, depending on their particular patterns of use, be diagnosed as having a substance dependency disorder, commonly referred to as addiction. Athletes can suffer from a number of other PDs including compulsive disorders, and a combination of alcohol and/or drug, and/or gambling, and/or sex problems are common in the lives of self-confessed sporting addicts. They are not unusual given that comorbidity is common among those with PDs. Orford (2011: 102) reports that there are consistent findings:

> . . . that gambling, alcohol consumption and drug taking are positively correlated and that gambling and other forms of addiction co-occur in the same people to a significantly greater degree than would be expected by chance.

Chronic addiction is often associated with other psychiatric conditions such as depression, panic disorder and phobia (Orford 2011; Pickard and Pearce 2013). Gogarty and Williamson (2009) provide an interesting analysis of the similar nature and source of some of these factors or 'demons', which they believe contributed to the problems of George Best, Diego Maradona and Paul Gascoigne. Difficult childhood experiences, family problems and narcissistic tendencies are common in the biographies of addicts, athletes and otherwise.

Alcoholism

According to Martin (2006: 89), alcoholism might take many forms, but generally speaking it can be described as 'long-term heavy involvement with alcohol in ways that lead to systematic loss of control and to significant problems – for example, by threatening goods such as health, safety, family, jobs and financial stability'. The definition and diagnosis of disorders in general, and alcohol-related disorder in particular, is complex, but a key reference point is the American Psychiatric Association's *Diagnostic and Statistical Manual of Mental Disorders* (DSM), which offers a standard classification and diagnostic criteria for a range of officially recognized disorders.[2] We are currently on the fifth version (DSM-5) and each incarnation sees new additions and deletions as certain conditions are formally recognized as disorders and others are removed. Cafri et al. (2008), for example, contributed to the identification and recognition of muscle dysmorphia, a type of body dismorphic disorder characterized by excessive pursuit of a muscular body. Prior to 1973, homosexuality was included as a disorder. Despite the DSM's influence, concerns remain about the danger of medicalizing moral or anti-social problems. According to Martin (2006), the DSM does not have the monopoly on defining disorders, but is very powerful nonetheless in shaping attitudes and policies towards behaviour that deviates from the norm. Being diagnosed with a 'disorder' has significant implications, not least in terms of access to medical services, health insurance and so on.

Talk of addiction is very different to the focus on character defects, vices or sin, which used to, and in some quarters continues to, provide the explanation for the phenomenon we now call alcoholism (or other substance abuse disorders). Terms like gluttony, intemperance, lack of self-control, lack of will power and so on fix the behaviour on a moral, rather than a medical, continuum. There continues to be a debate in the literature about the status of addiction as either a health or a moral issue. The distinction is potentially important for a number of reasons. If it is a health issue, an illness of the mind, a number of important ramifications in terms of how the person should be treated, follow. Generally speaking, we think of a person as suffering from an illness over which they have no control, whose cause is some kind of pathology and whose cure is some form of medical intervention. We are inclined to feel sorry for them and offer sympathy and assistance. If it is a defect of character or a vice we tend to judge and blame the individual and advocate some form of punishment (see previous chapter). According to Martin (2006), it was Alcoholics Anonymous (AA) that first brought the idea of alcohol disorder or alcoholism as an illness or disease into public consciousness. Formed in 1935 by two alcoholics, Bill Wilson and Dr Bob Smith, in Akron, Ohio, AA brought together a number of ideas about alcoholism and its treatment. The book, *Alcoholics Anonymous*, was published in 1939 and draws on medical, social, psychological and religious views about the causes of, and solutions to, alcoholism. It proposes many important ideas, not least the claim that the alcoholic's body is different; they are allergic to alcohol. In other words, alcoholism has an identifiable organic cause like other physical illnesses, and therefore is not merely a matter of weakness of will. Alcoholism is a sickness not a sin. Since its inception AA has had its supporters and detractors inside and outside the medical profession, and some of its claims, if taken literally, belie scientific evidence. Nevertheless, one of the central tenets, namely that alcoholism is a disease, has become received wisdom. The World Health Organization (WHO) sees the prevention and treatment of alcoholism and alcohol misuse as a key priority.

Alcoholism: a brain disease?

It seems that the motive to cleave disordered drinking behaviour from normal drinking behaviour, and to discover an underlying pathological cause for the former, is at least partly to do with its phenomenological characteristics. It feels or seems 'outside' of one's control. In Frankfurt's terms, the behaviour is a result of a will we wish we did not have. The inability to bring the behaviour under our conscious control, the fact that it is purportedly compulsive or compelled, means it shares features with other bodily illnesses that happen *to* us. No matter how hard I try, I cannot stop the blisters appearing when I burn my hand on a hot stove. Once the contact is made there is an inevitable biological chain of events beyond my control that manifests in observable symptoms. It seems that no matter how hard an addict tries, they cannot stop using alcohol or other substances. It therefore seems plausible to think that in the addict's case the 'body' must be doing something *to* them over which they have no control, generating an overwhelming compulsion or craving. According to Matthews (2007), the medical model of mental disorder (early proponents include AA) – that is, mental disorder as mental illness – is now the orthodoxy in Western medical/scientific culture.

> Mental illness, on this conception, is seen as parallel to bodily illness, as the latter is conceived in modern scientific medicine. [The medical model] . . . is understandably regarded as the only possible way for an enlightened person in a scientific culture to think of the bizarre, unintelligible, ways of thinking, acting, feeling, desiring and so on to which some of our fellow humans beings are subject . . . . They should not be stigmatized, but treated with sympathy, like other sufferers. Indeed, it is important on this view to see them as suffering from mental illness and its consequences, as patients, in the same way that those with bodily illnesses suffer from their conditions and their consequences. (Matthews 2007: 4)

Leshner (1997: 46) is unequivocal in calling addiction a brain disease:

> The addicted brain is distinctly different from non-addicted brain, as manifested by changes in brain metabolic activity, receptor availability, gene expression, and responsiveness to environmental cues.

The implication is that some form of pathology *causes* certain brain mechanisms to produce compulsive drinking. The addict is powerless over these mechanisms in the way indicated by Frankfurt above. If this is right, there are fundamental implications for the treatment of addiction. If the brain is the problem, then the brain would seem the obvious direct target for any medical intervention, as opposed to the agent. The treatment of some PDs already involves methods targeted at the brain such as the use of drugs like anti-depressants, surgery and electroconvulsive therapy. The success of drug treatments for conditions like schizophrenia 'lends force to the idea that mental disorder is an illness requiring medical treatment'

(Matthews 2007: 5) and that the effective treatment of all such disorders, including alcoholism, will eventually be a matter of treating the brain.[3] Such purported progress in putting addiction and brain disease on the same footing as other diseases, however, has not led (yet) to addicts and other PDs being treated like sufferers of other illnesses such as cancer. In terms of healthcare and the law addicts are *not* treated the same as other patients (Foddy 2010). They are denied disability benefits, and in many countries they might be jailed for using illegal drugs. The use of these drugs is a symptom of their illness. Moreover, not all PDs are treatable with pharmaceuticals, unless sedation counts as effective treatment.

So although the brain disease view is prevalent, it is by no means an uncontested or unproblematic one, in terms of description, diagnosis or treatment. Although the language of PD and mental illness turns away from the dated vocabulary of vice and sin and towards a 'medical' lexicon, cultural norms and values continue to play a key role in diagnosing and defining PD. Many disorders, including addiction, are not diagnosed by brain scans or blood tests or other diagnostic devices, but rather in terms of behaviour measured against criteria such as the DSM or some such. According to Pickard (2011a: 183), PDs to a greater or lesser extent are diagnosed 'via characteristics or traits that count as failures of morality or virtue and thus impair social, occupational, or other areas of interpersonal functioning'. Furthermore, the 'characteristics and traits that cause distress and impairment to the individual often involve harm to others' (Pickard 2011a: 182). It is the behaviour and its consequence to the individual and others around them that is at the centre of diagnosis, not the mechanisms underlying the behaviour.

From a theoretical/philosophical perspective, there are a number of difficulties in seeing PD like addiction as a form of (mental) illness or disease. The main difficulty is the role of choice. For Matthews (2007), being ill entails being in an undesirable state which was not chosen. People can become ill as a consequence of bad choices – for example, smoking – but the illness itself (cancer) was not chosen. 'Something can be an indirect consequence of a free choice without itself being freely chosen' (Matthews 2007: 120). Bodily illnesses are the outcome of causes such as infection, injury, the effects of chemicals or substances or some genetic factors: 'they are *external* to the sufferer, not within his or her conscious control' (Matthews 2007: 121). According to Matthews (2007), mental disorders are not best explained in such causal terms. They are choices, or the result of choices and these (bad) choices are best understood in terms of reasons rather than in terms of a dysfunction of the mind or brain. Granted they are abnormal or irrational, but choices none the less (Heyman 2013). Even though the behaviour deviates from the norm, PDs are *acting* in the full sense of the word; they are exercising their (disordered) agency. The view that addicts are agents rather than victims is reflected in our intuitions and in our legal and health systems. This is not to deny the science which points to identifiable brain-level processes or mechanisms that are implicated in disorder. Rather, it is to doubt the significance of such findings in its explanation. It does not follow that the identification of a brain process, even a faulty one, fully or even partly explains the disorder. There are brain processes behind every human behaviour and emotion, but we would not seek to explain an act of love or kindness in terms of the brain-level process that generated it. Advances in medical science will not solve this issue either. If we believe that addiction is a result of some organic pathology, in other words that an addict's compulsion is caused by the 'faulty' brain, this does not really tell us anything that most people do not already believe. It might narrow down the area of the brain or identify the genotype for addiction, but Morse (2011: 165) argues that: 'any black-box mechanical model of addiction would have done as well'. Foddy (2010: 26) argues that:

> Plasticity is a normal and largely beneficial characteristic of human brains, and thus if we made 'changes in brain structure and function' a sufficient criterion for disease we would define everyone as diseased.

What has to be shown, according to Foddy, is that the mechanism that causes the behaviour is different from mechanisms that cause behaviour in non-addicts. Morse (2011: 166) similarly argues that: 'Biological causation, even abnormal biological causation is not the equivalent of compulsion. If it were, all behaviour would be compelled'.

So why do we think the behaviour is compelled or caused? As has been discussed already, it seems to us, and feels to addicts, like their use is compulsive. Their judgement is immune to the negative consequences of using. Even potent and extreme disincentives which would sway 'normal' people, such as the health and well-being of one's children or the threat of jail, are not powerful enough to stop some addicts using. The threat of exposure, public humiliation, bankruptcy, disease or injury did not stop George Best from 'feeding' his addiction. It seems we infer that extremely irrational behaviour must be compelled, because we cannot make sense of it otherwise. If it is not, surely addicts would stop. Furthermore, addicts report or describe their use as compulsive and insist that they 'cannot help' using even though they may have a strong desire to stop. Flanagan (2011: 277) describes his own addiction in the following terms:

> The desire to live was not winning the battle over death. The overwhelming need – the pathological, unstoppable – need to use, was. Living was just a necessary condition of using.

There is another possible explanation. According to Aristotle (1980), pain and regret are evidence that an action is not *really* chosen. Regret implies that I did not want to do what I did, but somehow was not able to desist. Addicts sometimes regret their use and feel remorse for using. They are often sorry when their behaviour causes harm and promise not to do it again.

Neither explanation provides sufficient grounds for accepting that addicts are being acted upon against their will (Frankfurt 1971; Aristotle 1980) in a way which separates them from the rest of us. Foddy (2010) argues that non-addicted people share the characteristic of being immune to the cost of their behaviour. The behaviour is qualitatively different not categorically different. The adulterer, for example, will know that his actions are likely to cause significant pain and harm to himself and others if caught, yet he chooses to continue with his actions because he values the excitement and rewards of his behaviour (Tiger Woods' explanation for adultery was that he was addicted). Moreover, he may deeply regret his actions afterwards when things go wrong, but neither his immunity to reason nor his regret should count as evidence that he is *compelled* to cheat. According to Levy (2011), addicts do seem to be able to make rational choices even in relation to their drug/alcohol/behaviour and are able to abstain, sometimes for prolonged periods. In his autobiography, the footballer Tony Adams recalls abstaining for months in the lead up to an important tournament, but then going back to heavy drinking as soon as the tournament was over (Adams 1998: 12). Further evidence against the compulsive conclusion is that many addicts stop being addicts; they 'mature out' or give up without any interventions (Levy 2011: 92).[4] Moreover, interventions are based on the idea that change is possible and all psychotherapeutic interventions are predicated on the belief that addicts can be helped to change their behaviour.

Do addicts choose?

The evidence that addicts are compelled, therefore, is shaky. Does this mean that addicts are choosing their behaviour in the same way we might choose cereal over toast for breakfast? Given what has been said about PDs such as addiction, it seems counterintuitive to conclude that the behaviour is simply chosen in this way, even if the evidence that it is compelled is unreliable. According to Matthews (2007), part of the problem relates to our conception of human choice as the careful and rational weighing up of alternatives in light of our values or preferences. This is an overly simplified explanation that does not take into account the full complexity of personality and its development over time. As I discussed in Chapter 4, we develop dispositions and habits of emotion, thought, perception and action. Matthews (2007: 124) argues that:

> . . . an impulsive action is as much an expression of choice as one resulting from careful thought and deliberation. My impulses are surely as much part of me as my reflective thoughts: they are not imposed on me from the outside.

Impulses are different from reflexes in that they have an intentional object (drugs or some such) at which they are directed. An impulse to take drugs involves thoughts about a state of mind one would like to have and the understanding of how drugs will help achieve this.

> These are one's own thoughts, and so the decision comes from within oneself, not from outside, but the thought is not made conscious, and is not governed by generally accepted standards of rationality. (Matthews 2007: 124)

According to Matthews (2007), other intentional states are chosen in the sense that they are ours, such as our emotions, and need not be conscious in the strict sense mentioned above; that is, rational and careful deliberation at the time. Nevertheless, they are similarly intentional and directed and are as much chosen as other actions. The seemingly irrational compulsive actions of an addict can be thought of and understood in terms of (bad) choices broadly conceived. It is the same point that Aristotle (1980) makes about our habits. Actions that issue from them may be habitual; however, it does not mean they are not *my* actions or that it is something that happens *to* me.

Are addicts responsible?

When asking whether addicts are responsible, it might be helpful to be more precise about which specific aspects of their behaviour we are talking about. Flanagan (2011: 282) discusses two aspects of the addict's behaviour. The first, he calls 'addiction – 1', which describes the mental obsession (preoccupation with the substance) and physical compulsion to consume. It is this feature that neuroscientists and medics have attempted to describe and identify at the level of the brain. Levy (2011) calls this immediate and purportedly compulsive craving-driven consuming behaviour 'proximate'. It is characterized by an immediate and pressing need to fulfil a desire. The second feature of the addict's behaviour, 'addiction – 2', refers to addiction – 1 plus the addict's lifestyle, which includes 'characteristic situations, feelings, and behaviors associated with use, for example, various kinds of cues, preparatory rituals, behaviors, outcomes and so on' (Flanagan 2011: 282). This 'lifestyle' is a little broader, but includes what Levy (2011) calls 'distal' behaviour, namely the behaviour required to get hold of the drug, which varies according to its availability and legality. An alcoholic does not normally commit an offence in buying alcohol, whereas a heroin addict does when she buys heroin.

   When asking whether addicts are responsible we are asking at least three questions. The first has been discussed already: do addicts have any control over their compulsive use (addiction – 1)? The second is whether addicts are responsible for the harm caused to others as a result of their lifestyle (addiction – 2)? And, finally, are addicts responsible for becoming addicted? So, are addicts responsible for their lifestyle? It might be useful to narrow this down to a specific issue. Let us consider those addicts whose addiction has led them to neglect their children. They leave their children alone in the house to go out and get drunk.[5] Calum Best, George Best's son, recalls an incident when he came to visit his father in the UK. He had flown by himself from the USA and went with his father to a Manchester United FC game. After the game, George Best left his 11-year-old son alone in a hotel and went drinking, returning a day and a half later:

> At about 8 pm I come back to the table from one of my little football runs and my dad isn't there. He's gone, and so has everyone else, and I don't know what to do. I'm standing there with my ball, staring at the chairs where they were all sitting and looking around the lobby for my dad, but I can't see him. (Best 2015)

Even if we accept that George Best 'suffered' from an illness that compelled him to drink, it is difficult to accept that this exculpates him from a range of other responsibilities like attending to the well-being of his son. It is clear that, when drunk, decision-making capacity is severely compromised, and for some fatally so. According to Foddy (2010: 28):

> The brains of acutely intoxicated addicts, for example, are not capable of making the kinds of reliable judgments that are required for moral responsibility, according to every popular philosophical account.

Addicts often talk of doing things 'in blackout', a condition where they are acting, and moving around, but have no memory whatsoever of doing so (Jones 2014: 493). As I have mentioned, however, neither our moral intuitions nor the law look favourably on crimes committed when intoxicated, even during a blackout. As I discussed in the previous chapter, there is significant variation in how drunken offenders and victims are perceived depending on the nature of the offences. The reason that being drunk is generally not accepted as an excusing condition, even *if* we accept that when drunk the behaviour is not fully under the agent's control, is that we hold the agent responsible for getting drunk. Aristotle (1980: 60) argued that:

> Indeed we punish a man for his very ignorance, if he is thought responsible for the ignorance as when penalties are doubled in the case of drunkenness; for the moving principle is in the man himself, since he had the power of not getting drunk and his getting drunk was the cause of his ignorance.

In this chapter, however, I have been looking at those special cases where individuals are addicted and allegedly 'cannot help' getting drunk. Even if we accept the theory, and I have presented strong arguments against it, that there are compulsive causes outside the alcoholic's control, Morse (2011: 179–180), echoing Matthews' (2007) earlier observations, argues that this does not necessarily get the alcoholic 'off the hook':

> Compulsive states are marked by allegedly overwhelming desires or cravings, but whether the cravings are produced by faulty biology, including genetic predispositions or neural defects, faulty psychology, faulty environment, or some combination of the three, a desire is just a desire, and its satisfaction by seeking and using is human action . . . . The addict desires, broadly, either the pleasure of intoxication, the avoidance of the pain of withdrawal or inner tension or both. The addict believes that using the substance will satisfy the desire and consequently forms the intention to seek and use the substance.

If both Morse and Matthews are right, then an addict is responsible for getting drunk and it is reasonable to hold them equally accountable for their actions when drunk as we do non-addicts. There may of course be reasons to treat them differently, but I will return to this later.

The final question was whether the addict is responsible for becoming an addict, although this might not be so important given the preceding conclusion. For the sake of argument, if it is true that the addict can no longer choose whether they can abstain (they have developed a habit), there was a point in the past, before they became addicted, when they could. Their first use must be considered an autonomous choice in the normal sense of the term. The idea of 'tracing', discussed in the previous chapter, is pertinent here. Recall that tracing is the idea that even if we establish that the offender is not responsible now (because he is drunk) and claim that he is incapable of not getting drunk (because he is an addict), we can still ask the further question; is he responsible for becoming an addict? Again, Aristotle (1980: 61) is insightful here:

> We may suppose a case in which he was ill voluntarily, through living incontinently and disobeying his doctors. In that case it was *then* open to him not to be ill, but now, when he has thrown away his chance, just as when you have let a stone go it is too late to recover it; but yet it was in your power to throw it, since the moving principle was in you. So, too, to the unjust and the self-indulgent man it was open at the beginning not to become men of this kind, and so they are unjust and self-indulgent voluntarily; but now that they have become so it is not possible for them not to be so.

Morse (2011), like Aristotle, believes that an addict is responsible for becoming addicted. The reasons for concluding thus are generally persuasive; becoming addicted involves a series of choices including taking the first drink, cigarette or drug. The risks associated with heroin and tobacco are well documented and well publicized. Individuals who choose to experiment and repeat the choice despite the warnings are surely culpable in their own fate.

There are two points to make here. First, this argument is *prima facie* persuasive, but only if we take an oversimplified view of addiction. People become addicted by repeated and incremental use of a substance, a series of discrete voluntary actions. The medical model tells us that such use will change the brain in some important way and cause addiction. However, only some individuals who experiment with addictive substances become addicts. According to Morse (2011: 176), it is between 15 and 17%. There are many purported contributory factors at play in addition to the consumption of the substance. These include genetic predisposition, personality type, up-bringing and social and economic circumstances, which impact the chances of becoming addicted (see Jones 2015: 10; Gogarty and Williamson 2009). There seems to be an identifiable at-risk group of people. According to Pickard and Pearce (2013) those who go on to become chronic long-term addicts are likely to suffer from other psychological conditions whereas most people who qualify as substance dependent mature out without clinical intervention. Many can and do use psychoactive substances without the attendant problems associated with addiction.

Second, even for those at risk, addiction does not occur unless there is repeated use of the substance or behaviour, although some claim that they became 'hooked' immediately. People usually experiment with addictive substances like alcohol and drugs around mid to late adolescence (Morse 2011). Although this age group are not fully developed in terms of rational capacity and evidence suggests that they have a higher propensity for risk-taking, Morse argues that they are capable of making rational decisions about the risks associated with drugs. Furthermore, he argues there is sufficient information available to conclude that 'those who take drugs understand the risks sufficiently to be held responsible if addiction ensues' (Morse 2011: 176). In relation to alcohol, however, the picture is not so clear-cut. Throughout this book, I have drawn attention to a number of differences between alcohol and other drugs. Such differences are writ large in this context. One might reasonably ask, given the facts about alcohol use in society discussed previously, whether Morse's conclusion is justified in relation to alcohol. The messages about potential addiction risks to alcohol are virtually non-existent in comparison to the positive promotion and normalization of alcohol. Moreover, at-risk individuals are unlikely to be aware that they are especially at risk at the time they experiment. Even if they are aware of certain risk factors, for example they know one of their parents was alcoholic, they might be unwilling either to recognize their increased risk or change their behaviour in light of these risks. Calum Best's experience is interesting. His grandmother and father were both alcoholics, yet he experimented, and had problems with, alcohol and other drugs despite being concerned that he might follow in his father's footsteps. In his auto-biography he writes: 'The fact that I'm drunk most of the time is messing with my emotions, and I'm a mess' (Best 2015: 233–234). It seems that he has now been able to straighten himself out, but his life was, and perhaps remains, characterized by a number of the personality and behavioural aspects associated with addic-tion. Knowing about the factors that predispose addiction ought not change how alcoholics should be treated in terms of moral and legal responsibility, but there is a clear message here in terms of education, prevention and care, especially in relation to individuals who are showing signs of problems at a young age.

A further issue about the addict's responsibility for their condition relates to their continued addiction. Paul Gascoigne, the former professional football player, has been aware for a number of years that he has a problem with alcohol. Countless treatments at the world's leading rehabilitation centres have been followed by an inevitable relapse and associated problems. Even if he did not know he was to become an addict when he started drinking, he knows it now, and we might rightly argue that he has a responsibility to do something about it. The combination of a culture which normalizes alcohol use, celebrates and condones drunken escapades, and is largely ignorant to the causes and conditions of addiction, may also make it difficult for those seeking to give up alcohol to do so. George Best famously never managed it. Why some do and some do not manage to recover is a question beyond this book, but it seems that the desire to stop is an important prerequisite.

To summarize the chapter so far, being an addict should not provide a *general* reason why one should not be held responsible for one's lifestyle, harmful behaviours and offences. Even if an offence is committed in 'a state of uncon-sciousness or blackout induced by substance use' (Morse 2011: 190), addicts are held accountable both for getting into such a state and for becoming addicts. Nevertheless, addiction is a complex phenomenon with a number of social, psychological and neurological antecedents and certain individuals are at greater risk of addiction for reasons that are beyond their control.

Addicted athletes?

So far, I have discussed the concept of addiction and its implications in the abstract. What does all this mean for athletes, clubs, governing bodies, and coaches? There are two issues I want to address. The first is about how we should treat athletes who have a substance abuse disorder or alcoholism, and the second but closely related question is about who decides or diagnoses the condition.

Punishment or therapy

The discussion above focuses on whether an addict is responsible for their actions and there are two ways the issue could go. The first is that the addict is ill and not responsible, with the implication that they should not be punished. The second is that the addict is responsible and should be as accountable for his or her actions as a non–addict. At this stage of the chapter I want to further problematize the idea that addicts must either be ill and not responsible, or not ill and therefore fully responsible. Such a dichotomy, sometimes expressed in terms of a medical versus a moral model, neither paints an accurate picture of the complexity of addiction nor is helpful when it comes to dealing with addicts. Martin (2006) believes that it is unhelpful to think of addiction as *either* a medical issue *or* a moral issue. Matthews (2007) believes that it is similarly unhelpful to think that we should either punish *or* treat addicts.

Deciding if someone has a problem is not an exact science. If they are showing signs of abusing alcohol they might benefit from some form of therapy to help them change their behaviour. This need not be instead of punishment, but alongside punishment. Addicted prisoners are required to attend treatment programmes while incarcerated. According to Matthews (2007: 162), 'such programmes are both punishment, in that they are unwelcome to the offender, and also treatment in that they are therapy for the condition which gives rise to the offence'. The balance is a tricky one to achieve, however, because for therapy to be effective, talking therapies in particular, the individual has to cooperate with the process. This cooperation often comes only after what alcoholics describe as 'a moment of clarity' or when they have hit 'rock bottom', recognition that they have had enough and have developed 'a desire to change' (Babor et al. 2010: 221). Sugar Ray Leonard recalls such a moment in his autobiography:

> For years, I ran – to the gym, to cocaine, to the bottle, to other women, to anything or anyone that would make the pain disappear, which it did, though never for long.

That July, I finally stopped running. I looked at my eyes in the mirror, just as I did in the dressing room before my toughest fights. What I saw I had never seen before, my eyes willing to admit I needed help, and before it was too late. (Leonard 2011: 291)

I believe that athletes whose offending might be symptomatic of addiction should both be held accountable for the offence, but also receive help. According to Pickard (2011a), it is an important part of the therapeutic process that the service user is encouraged to take responsibility for their actions, which may include accepting punishment for any offences they commit as a result of their addictive lifestyle or being intoxicated. They should not be let off the hook regardless of whether they meant it, had control over it and so on. Treating or helping addicts is predicated on the notion that they can choose to change. Addicts can, with help, regain some control over the behaviour which is causing problems; otherwise there would be no point in offering help. Treatment requires addicts to take responsibility for their behaviour and be committed to learn to choose and act otherwise (Pickard 2011b: 210).

Currently, there seems to be a very mixed picture of the way athletes are treated. Depending on which country the athlete is in, their sport, performance level, the nature of the offence and the symptoms displayed, there may be a very different approach. Earlier in the book I mentioned the case of Matt Stevens, an English rugby union player who tested positive for cocaine, and the English cricketer, Tom Maynard, whose post mortem revealed systematic cocaine use. It seems that cocaine use immediately raises concerns about addiction. It is a red flag! We think that cocaine users need help because they are thought to be on a path to addiction, or already there. They must stop or their life will be inevitably ruined. Matt Stevens did seek help while serving his 2 year anti-doping ban. Seeking treatment, however, was not a condition or a requirement of returning to the game. Alcohol is very different. In the UK, athletes, or anyone else for that matter, who drink and drive or get into fights because of alcohol are not normally expected to seek help for alcohol issues. Their behaviour is not necessarily at odds with the ethos as discussed in Chapter 4. Doing stupid things when drunk is not a red flag; in fact it is sometimes a badge of honour. At times athletes who have been violent when drunk are advised to get help with 'anger management', which for addicts is, according to Gogarty and Williamson (2009: 35), 'the psychological equivalent of putting a plaster on a severed artery'. In the USA, the picture is different. It is far more likely that an elite athlete who offends in relation to alcohol will be required to undertake some form of treatment and may even be required to abstain from alcohol as part of a formal agreement. This is in addition to, or as part of, being punished. The National Hockey League (NHL), for example, has a well-established substance abuse programme which, among other things, stipulates what is required of players who are deemed to have committed alcohol and other drug-related offences. The programme is seen as:

> ... a comprehensive effort to address substance abuse among NHL players and their families, to treat those with a substance abuse problem in a confidential, fair and effective way, and to deter such abuse in future. The program seeks to accomplish these goals through a coordinated program of education, counselling, inpatient and outpatient treatment, follow up care, and, where appropriate, sanctions.[6]

It is a blend of education, therapy and punishment, designed to help the athlete tackle any problem they might have, but also to try and protect the NHL's valuable assets and reputation. Once an athlete is registered, they are required to fulfil certain obligations and a failure to do so can lead to increased punishment (for example, suspension from play) and/or further engagement with the programme. This is a compulsory scheme to which athletes have to adhere. The National Football League (NFL) has a similar programme, and recently Denver Broncos' Matt Prater was suspended for four games for violating the substance abuse policy. Having been put in the programme for driving under the influence in 2011, he was banned because he had 'a couple of beers' on holiday, which constituted an infringement of the programme.[7] In the UK the approach is different. In football, if an athlete offends and alcohol was involved they may be suspended by their club or the national team, or both, but there is no compulsory treatment element to the punishment. The Professional Footballers' Association (PFA) offers support, advice and education, and funds treatment for both current and former players in a rehabilitation centre for various disorders including alcoholism. This is a voluntary service often accessed after their career has come to an end. If we accept that there are such conditions as addiction, and that such conditions genuinely contribute to problematic behaviour, then it seems right and compassionate that treatment (or help) as well as punishment are available for addicts or potential addicts (whatever that might mean).

Diagnosis

If we accept that both punishment and therapy are preferable, further key issues arise in terms of diagnosis. I mentioned above that despite advances in brain science, addictions like alcoholism are diagnosed by a psychiatrist, psychotherapist or other health professional, via the behaviour of the individual. A standard test such as the Alcohol Use Disorders Test (AUDIT), developed by the WHO, might be used.[8] This test consists of 10 questions designed to test whether an individual is an alcoholic, and includes questions such as:

- how often do you have six or more drinks on one occasion (this is equivalent to six 330 ml bottles of 5% beer or 4 pints of 4% beer)?
- how often do you have a drink containing alcohol?
- how often during the past year have you felt guilty or remorseful after drinking?
- how often in the last year have you been unable to remember what happened the night before because you had been drinking?
- have you or someone else been injured as a result of your drinking?

- how often during the last year have you failed to do what was normally expected of you because of drinking?
- has a relative or friend or a doctor or another health worker been concerned about your drinking or suggested you cut down?

Alcoholics Anonymous (AA) also has a set of questions, but none focus on quantity or frequency of drinking; rather, the focus is on the effect or impact that drinking has. For example, they ask:

- has your drinking caused trouble at home?
- do you tell yourself you can stop drinking any time you want to, even though you keep getting drunk when you don't mean to?
- do you envy people who can drink without getting into trouble?
- have you missed days off work because of drinking?
- do you ever try to get 'extra' drinks at a party because you do not get enough?
- have you decided to stop drinking for a week or so, but only lasted a couple of days?[9]

Theo Fleury's drinking career was certainly characterized by many, if not all, of these elements. In one particular passage he describes how one drink led to another and to another and:

> I went on a good drunk for a few days. I started out at a bar, and when it closed I found a buddy's place. I drank everything in his house – beer, whisky, whatever. Then back to the bar. I kept it up thanks to a little help from cocaine and marijuana. It took me four or five days with no sleep to get the loss out of my system. This became standard procedure for me at the end of every year. I set my record for consecutive days partying in 1998, when I stayed up for the entire Calgary Stampede – that's ten days. (Fleury 2009: 95)

To an extent diagnosis is self-diagnosis. An individual has to decide for themselves whether they have a problem, perhaps by answering such questions above honestly. They have to accept there is a problem and that problem is alcohol rather than stress, anger, boredom or some such. Following this acceptance they must have the desire and willingness to change. Calum Best feels his father never really had the desire to change. Even after a liver transplant, and when dying in hospital, George Best continued to drink. 'He [the doctor] is doing everything he can, but my dad isn't really helping them. When he gets the chance, which is any time he's able to leave the hospital, he's drinking' (Best 2015: 177). This willingness to admit or recognize a problem may of course develop as part of the therapeutic journey, and an unwilling participant may come to accept or recognize that they have a problem as the process unfolds. Equally, they may not. I am not a therapist or health practitioner so I will not delve any deeper into issues relating to therapeutic effectiveness; however, if conditions like addiction are real, their reality is not in the eye of the beholder, so to speak. They can be diagnosed, but perhaps not treated, independently of a subject's agreement. Moreover, they can persist/exist independently of either formal (clinical) diagnosis or self-diagnosis. When the disorder is in its infancy or developing, it might not be so easy to identify behaviour as symptoms of a potential disorder. In a culture where binge drinking is the norm, the potential addict does not stand out (see Chapter 3). Their behaviour may become more obviously problematic as they get older and their drinking problem gets worse, but at an early stage it might be put down to immaturity, being a 'party animal', not being able to hold their drink or a range of other rationalizations. In this respect alcoholism is very different to other bodily illnesses or diseases where there are often clear and indubitable symptoms and diagnostic tests. The parent whose child comes home drunk rarely worries about addiction, whereas the parent whose child experiments with heroin will be extremely concerned.

D'Angelo and Tamburrini (2010) invite us to consider doping offences as potentially symptomatic of early or potential addiction. In other words, athletes who dope are at risk of becoming addicts. Consequently, they argue that dopers 'should be handled in accordance with that characterization' (D'Angelo and Tamburrini 2010: 700) and be offered treatment and therapy rather than being ostracized from the athletic community. I am not wholly persuaded by their argument in relation to performance-enhancing drugs (see Jones 2015), but one might make a more persuasive case along these lines in relation to alcohol. As we have seen, getting into trouble while drunk is 'red flag' for alcohol-related problems for a number of elite sport organizations in the USA.

Let us consider a hypothetical case study. An elite male professional athlete gets very drunk as part of an extended celebration, organized and endorsed by the coaching and management team. Free alcohol is provided by sponsors and many of the players and coaches drink heavily as is normal in such occasions. This player, however, gets very drunk and loses self-control and is arrested in the early hours of the following morning for fighting. Passers by photograph him, clearly intoxicated, in a struggle with police. The story and his picture make the media headlines the following day. This is not the first time the player has been involved in such an incident. He has been involved in a few other incidents that have come to the public's attention and has been reprimanded and punished in the past. Nevertheless, he is fit and in good condition and performs to a high standard on the pitch. The player has committed an offence against the disciplinary rules set down by the team. As discussed in the previous chapter, punishment gives a clear signal to the player that the behaviour is bad, and the severity of the punishment serves as a barometer for how bad. Punishment also deters others from engaging in similar behaviour. For Matthews (2007), punishing for these reasons is primarily aimed at the well-being of people other than the offender; that is, for the well-being of society as a whole. It sends a message that the behaviour is unacceptable. Nevertheless, punishment may also aim at reforming or rehabilitating the individual. The athlete who gets banned from playing should be less likely to offend again given the negative experience of losing playing time and salary, and the possible shame associated with the punishment. In this case, let us suppose that each incident is met with increasingly severe punishment, but it is not been effective (so far) at deterring the behaviour. The repetitive behaviour is causing the individual harm, but they seem incapable of changing or desisting. Their behaviour is potentially symptomatic of a developing problem because it manifests a number of elements listed above. They are not, however, exhibiting traits associated with chronic alcoholism (and may never do so). The question is, what should be done?

Orford (2011) argues that the development of addiction is a process that involves several stages. The first stage is taking an interest in alcohol. In Chapter 3, I argued that participation in (certain) sports may encourage or increase the chance of developing an interest in alcohol through a range of mechanisms. The next stage is experimenting with alcohol, and again this might happen with other team members with or without the encouragement and blessing of coaches or older players. Following this stage there may be further stages where the use becomes misuse or abuse and graduates to full-blown addiction. Different individuals might be vulnerable in different ways here. I have mentioned factors like genetic predisposition, but personality types, background and personal circumstance may all contribute. For example, a significant life event such as bereavement, serious injury or success might trigger an escalation of drinking. Theo Fleury believes his abuse at the hands of a hockey coach was pivotal: 'The direct result of my being abused was that I became a fucking raging alcoholic lunatic' (Fleury 2009: 27). Other predictors of problem alcohol use are childhood or adolescent behaviours characterized by impulsivity, aggression and being anti-social (Orford 2011: 103). According to Pickard and Pearce (2013), substance disorder is at its height in adolescence and early adulthood and the majority who abuse alcohol at this stage in their lives 'mature out' by the time they are around 30 years old without any clinical intervention. A minority, however, don't mature out and are not affected by punishment. They become long-term chronic addicts or their abuse becomes so bad that they require or seek help at a comparatively young age. This latter group are more likely to have another PD that complicates and exacerbates their drinking problems. It is not easy to decide which behaviours (and at which stage) constitute symptoms of addiction or potential addiction.

Alcoholism manifests itself in a variety of ways and may progress and develop differently in different people. Theo Fleury (in ice hockey) and Paul McGrath (in football) both recall playing matches while drunk and performing extremely well, not what we would readily associate with alcoholism. Mike Tyson was undisputed world champion while in the grip of numerous addictions, including alcohol. The key issue in diagnosing a disorder like alcoholism is not whether the individual is drunk all the time, but the effect drinking has, how it makes them behave and how they feel or interact with the substance in terms of their obsession or preoccupation with it. Moreover, there may be a host of other 'red flag' characteristics. In Paul Gascoigne's case, there was a catalogue of reckless defiant behaviour and a number of obsessions and compulsions including the fear of flying and overeating (he suffered from a number of other PDs that put him at further risk of addiction). So when athletes get into trouble when drunk this may be indicative of a deeper issue and a more significant problem. The point is that the use of alcohol alone is not a reliable indicator, particularly given the alcohol ethos discussed previously.

Athletes who offend where excessive alcohol is involved should be punished. If they offend again it is clear the deterrent effect of punishment has not worked. Some would argue that the punishment was not severe enough. We have seen that in North America governing bodies like the NHL prescribe therapeutic intervention in addition to punishment. There is evidence that a variety of brief interventions such as motivational interviewing (MI) are effective in reducing both risky alcohol consumption and alcohol-related problems (Wutzke et al. 2001). Vasilaki et al. (2006: 333) argue that MI 'is an effective intervention for reducing alcohol consumption', particularly with young adults who do not have severe drinking problems. Such interventions might help first offenders to control their drinking. Relevant sporting authorities, governing bodies and clubs should consider routinely providing support in conjunction with punishment. If these early interventions work for some individuals then they and other may be spared further problems and difficulties associated with their alcohol use. If they don't and the behaviour continues, as in the example above, this may be symptomatic of deeper-lying problems that require more comprehensive and intensive therapeutic intervention. There is of course, no guarantee that such therapy will work.

Compulsory therapy

One last important question I want to briefly examine is whether compulsory therapy is justifiable. The question of therapy only becomes relevant if we accept that some offences are the result of an underlying disorder such as addiction, and we can obtain a reliable diagnosis of the condition. Notwithstanding the potential efficacy issues of compulsory therapy, the decision to compel athletes, or anyone else for that matter, to have treatment is controversial. We have seen that diagnosis relies upon the individual openly and honestly admitting to their symptoms, but this is not always forthcoming. Denial, or a distorted thinking, is a common symptom of alcoholism and other addictions; therefore the athlete might not accept that they have a problem for which they are being given compulsory treatment. They may be treated without their consent or against their will. According to Matthews (2007: 164): 'One of the cornerstones of liberal medical ethics is that doctors must respect the autonomy of their patients'. The patient has the right to self-determination and may refuse treatment even if there is strong evidence that it would be in their best interest to accept it. In relation to mental illness, however, individuals are sometimes 'treated' against their will. In 2014, Paul Gascoigne was sectioned (again) under the Mental Health Act (government legislation in the UK which allows people to be detained against their will at the request of an approved mental health practitioner[10]) and was taken to a hospital for detoxification.[11] The practice is controversial because it means that the desires of individuals with mental disorders may be ignored.

The practice of compelling athletes to undertake treatment for alcohol problems similarly ignores the wishes or rights of athletes to make autonomous judgements and choices. Assuming that the reasons for insisting on therapy relate to the athlete's well-being, acting paternalistically to bring this about is controversial for many reasons. The issue of diagnosis, as has been mentioned above, is controversial. The powers to detain under the Mental Health Act are only enacted in extreme cases where the immediate well-being of an individual or others is at significant risk; in other words, the behaviour is extremely disordered or unpredictable. Moreover, an approved mental health practitioner has to make a judgement about the mental stability of the individual in question. The compulsory treatment of athletes raises a number of questions. They may not accept that they have a drink problem or a 'real' disorder, but are nevertheless forced to undertake a course of therapy or brief intervention regardless. The passage of time may or may not vindicate their view, it's impossible to know. Someone (employer, manager, coach and so on) has to decide that in light of their current behaviour an athlete should undergo some kind of therapeutic intervention. This decision might be enacted in light of a general rule or guideline that is set out in an athlete's contract and may or may not involve a diagnostic element. The athletes can choose not to attend therapy, but this will have significant implications for their contracts.

The paternalistic decision to compel individuals with (or with potential symptoms of) alcoholism to undergo treatment assumes that they are not competent to make the right decision. According to Matthews (2007), the idea of competence in relation to mental health is complex, both philosophically in terms of how we define it and in relation to which norms and criteria, and empirically in terms of how we decide that this particular individual is competent. Given the extensive discussion above about whether addicts have control, it is controversial to suggest that they do not have the competence to make important decisions about their own well-being. Other grounds for paternalistic action on behalf of addicts, such as their irrationality, or that they do not *really* know what they want, are similarly controversial. In extreme cases, where an individual is clearly in danger or risks endangering others, compelling them against their will seems justified. It is less easy to justify compelling individuals whose alcohol-related behaviour, may or may not be symptomatic of more deep seated problems. This raises a question about an elite athlete's rights in light of the conditions and obligations that form part of their contracts. If the alcohol ethos was different and we more readily accepted that abusing alcohol was a problem for which some need help, compulsory therapy might not be necessary. Individuals might recognize sooner that alcohol was an issue for them and seek help.

Summary

With some notable exceptions, I believe that problematic alcohol use in sport and society is not taken seriously. The behaviour is normalized and alcohol *misuse* in many contexts is considered *normal* alcohol use. In some subcultures, and at certain times, bad behaviour as a result of intoxication is par for the course. Certain individuals might be deterred by punishment, but others might continue to misuse or abuse alcohol and progress to suffer from chronic alcoholism. This is a genuine issue which punishment by itself will not resolve. Punishment, if an offence has occurred, *and* therapy, might be necessary and justified, but compulsory therapy raises a number of questions about the ethics and effectiveness of non-voluntary treatment. These issues may be exacerbated when the individual does not believe they have a problem with alcohol. Alcohol addiction, like many PDs, is a complex, multi-faceted phenomenon which involves much more than the compulsion to drink. Drink is often one symptom or condition among wider personality and behavioural issues which themselves are a manifestation of deep-seated habits and traits. In the next chapter I examine some of these broader personality and circumstantial issues associated with chronic alcoholism in more detail through the life story of a former professional footballer in the UK who suffered, but is now in recovery, from alcoholism.

Notes

1 See Tyson's (2013) and Leonard's (2011) autobiographies for the graphic and often disturbing extent of their disordered sex-related behaviour.
2 http://www.psychiatry.org/practice/dsm (accessed 6/02/2015).
3 In Finland, the standard treatment for alcohol dependence is the 'Sinclair method', which is a drug-based treatment that targets receptors in the brain to stop cravings. http://en.wikipedia.org/wiki/Sinclair_Method (accessed 25/02/2015).
4 Heyman (2013) makes similar claims that most addicts quit by themselves, but these are controversial to say the least. Dawson et al. (2006) found that for many alcoholics formal treatment and twelve-step recovery programmes were necessary. I am not sure how proponents of the 'maturing out' view would distinguish between the addicts who do mature out, and those who do not.
5 Recently, there have been a series of stories about addicted parents who have neglected their children in the most heinous ways, including letting them live in inhumane conditions without food, water or clean clothes.
6 http://sportsdocuments.com/2013/07/29/nhl-substance-abuse-program/ (accessed 12/03/2015).
7 http://www.sbnation.com/nfl/2014/8/24/6062315/denver-broncos-matt-prater-suspension (accessed 19/05/2015).
8 http://www.who.int/substance_abuse/activities/sbi/en/ (accessed 30/04/2015).
9 http://www.alcoholics-anonymous.org.uk/About-AA/Newcomers/Is-AA-for-you? (accessed 30/04/2015).
10 http://www.mind.org.uk/information-support/legal-rights/mental-health-act/?gclid=CJCniOr1osQCFWbKtAodIQQAhw#.VQGXX_msV8G (accessed 12/03/2015).
11 http://www.independent.co.uk/sport/football/news-and-comment/tottenham-offering-support-to-paul-gascoigne-amid-reports-of-former-england-midfielder-being-sectioned-9817829.html (accessed 12/03/2015).

References

Adams, T., 1998. *Addicted*. London: Collins Willow.
Aristotle, 1980. *The Nicomachean ethics.* Trans. W.D. Ross. Updated J.L. Ackrill and J.O. Urmsom. Oxford: Oxford University Press.
Babor, T., et al., 2010. *Alcohol: no ordinary commodity—research and public policy*, 2nd edn. Oxford: Oxford University Press.
Best, C., 2015. *Second Best: my dad and me*. London: Bantam Press.

Cafri, G., Olivardia, R. and Thompson, J.K., 2008. Symptom characteristics and psychiatric comorbidity among males with muscle dysmorphia. *Comprehensive Psychiatry*, 49, 374–379.

D'Angelo, C. and Tamburrini, C., 2010. Addict to win? A different approach to doping. *Journal of Medical Ethics*, 36, 700–707.

Dawson, D.A., et al., 2006. Estimating the effect of help-seeking on achieving recovery from alcohol dependence. *Addiction*, 101, 824–834.

Flanagan, O., 2011. What is it like to be an addict? In: J. Poland and G. Graham, eds. *Addiction and responsibility*. Cambridge, MA: MIT Press, 269–292.

Fleury, T., 2009. *Playing with fire*. Chicago, IL: Triumph Books.

Foddy, B., 2010. Addiction and its sciences – philosophy. *Addiction*, 106(1), 25–31.

Frankfurt, H., 1971. Freedom of the will and the concept of a person. *Journal of Philosophy*, 68(1), 5–20.

Gogarty, P. and Williamson, I., 2009. *Winning at all costs: sporting gods and their demons*. London: JR Books.

Heyman, G.M., 2013. Addiction and choice: theory and new data. *Frontiers in Psychiatry*, 4, 1–4.

Jones, C., 2014. Alcoholism and recovery: a case study of a former professional footballer. *International Review for the Sociology of Sport*, 49(3/4), 485–505.

Jones, C., 2015. Doping as addiction: disorder and moral responsibility. *Journal of the Philosophy of Sport*, 42(2), 251–267.

Leonard, S.R., 2011. *The big fight: my autobiography*. London: Ebury Press.

Leshner, A.I., 1997. Addiction is a brain disease, and it matters. *Science*, 278(45), 45–47.

Levy, N., 2011. Addiction, responsibility, and ego depletion. In: J. Poland and G. Graham, eds. *Addiction and responsibility*. Cambridge, MA: MIT Press, 89–111.

Martin, M.W., 2006. *From morality to mental health: virtue and vice in a therapeutic culture*. New York: Oxford University Press.

Matthews, E., 2007. *Body-subjects and disordered minds: treating the whole person in psychiatry*. Oxford: Oxford University Press.

Morse, S.J., 2011. Addiction and criminal responsibility. In: J. Poland and G. Graham, eds. *Addiction and responsibility*. Cambridge, MA: MIT Press, 159–199.

Orford, J., 2011. *An unsafe bet? The dangerous rise of gambling and the debate we should be having*. Chichester: Wiley-Blackwell.

Pickard, H., 2011a. What is personality disorder? *Philosophy, Psychiatry and Psychology*, 18(3), 181–184.

Pickard, H. 2011b. Responsibility without blame: empathy and the effective treatment of personality disorder. *Philosophy, Psychiatry and Psychology*, 18(3), 209–223.

Tyson, M., 2013. *Undisputed truth: my autobiography*. London: Harper Collins.

Vasilaki, E.I., Hosier, S.G. and Cox, W.M., 2006. The efficacy of motivational interviewing as a brief intervention for excessive drinking: a meta-analytic review. *Alcohol and Alcoholism*, 42(3), 328–335.

Wutzke, S.E., et al., 2001. Cost effectiveness of brief interventions for reducing alcohol consumption. *Social Science and Medicine*, 52, 863–887.

7 Footballer and alcoholic

A life story

Introduction

I have argued throughout this book for a change in attitude towards alcohol. It is a toxic substance that poses a number of risks for the consumer and to society. In the previous chapter I discussed the issue of alcohol-related personality disorder or addiction. It seems that some individuals may be particularly at risk of becoming addicted because of a complex blend of personal and social circumstances. Spotting the warning signs is not easy and, unlike other drugs, alcohol use, even excessive alcohol use, especially binge drinking, is not an immediate 'red flag' for addiction. As I have said, only a small percentage of those who use alcohol go on to become addicts, although excessive users may damage themselves and others in many ways. My aim in this chapter is to provide an insight into what being an alcoholic is like from the perspective of the addict. In order to do this I present a life story of a recovering alcoholic who had a brief, but ultimately unsuccessful, career in professional football in the UK. Part of my aim here is to provide a counterpoint to the playboy, party-going, free-spirited and glamorous narrative associated with some rich and famous addicted athletes and reveal some of the darker aspects of addiction.

A phenomenology of addiction

Owen Flanagan is a successful and well-known philosophy professor who specializes in the philosophy of mind, among other things. He is also recovering from an alcohol and prescription drug addiction. He attempts to give a philosophically informed account of what addiction is like, a first-person perspective of the phenomenon of addiction (Flanagan 2011). There is much more to his chapter than I can cover here, so I will select some of what I think are the most pertinent ideas to act as a foreground the life history that follows. Flanagan (2011: 270) describes addiction as a bewildering phenomenon which has the following structure:

> I wanted not to use, I expressed to myself, my loved ones, and to mental health professionals a sincere desire not to use, and I used. Again and again.

Flanagan recalls his first taste of alcohol. There was nothing particularly unusual about the occasion. He was in his early teens at his friend's house and they drank some hard apple cider. He has powerful recollections of what the apple cider did to him.

> I felt release from being scared and anxious. It was good. I did not know, I would not have known to say if asked at the time, that I was a scared and anxious type. Perhaps I did not know until that medicinal moment what it was like not to be scared and anxious. It is too long ago to say. However, it seems that at that moment on the corner of Secor Road and Hartsdale Avenue, a certain eighth-grade boy was released for a little time from a certain inchoate fear and anxiety. I loved this first drink. It calmed my soul. (Flanagan 2011: 275)

Not all addicts become addicted to substances which produce the feelings of safety that Flanagan chased. The feelings they chase are heterogeneous and the substance and processes addicts use to produce these feelings differ. Addicts may use or try other drugs and behaviours when their drug of choice is not available (for example, sex, gambling, food, tobacco, pornography, cocaine and prescription drugs all feature in the various stories of addicted athletes). Flanagan describes how his using eventually came to dominate everything and that he would need alcohol in the morning just to feel okay.

> The story about the beginning and the end of my drinking career seems to have a simple experiential logical structure: I found some substance that alleviated a certain inchoate fear. I liked that substance, or better, I liked its effect; I used it. Eventually it produced a much worse dreadfulness than the fear it initially provided relief from. But by then I couldn't find my way to stop. (Flanagan 2011: 278)

For non-addicts, the behaviour of addicts is bewildering and it is difficult to understand and empathize with them. At least part of this problem relates to the general issue in philosophy of 'other minds' and access to them. Flanagan (2011: 281), following Nagel (1979), argues that there 'is something that it is like' to have conscious experience which is true for each person. Knowing what 'it is like for you', having knowledge about your experience (as opposed to mine), however, is a complex issue. Many people have experienced being drunk, but being an addict, Flanagan (2011: 282) argues, is not like being drunk all the time, even though it does involve being drunk a lot.

> What it is like to be an addict involves both more and less than being drunk or high all the time. It involves more than this because addiction involves constant self-loathing that being drunk needn't involve. And it involves less than being wasted all the time because much of the activity of middle and late addiction involves maintenance dosing.

There are a number of theories about the nature and cause of addiction including psychological, sociological and neuropsychological explanations, but they are not capable of telling us what it is like to be an addict: 'Only the individual organism is situated to *have* its own experiences' (Flanagan 2011: 283). In the previous chapter, I mentioned Flanagan's description of two broad categories of addictive experience (addiction – 1 and addiction – 2). The first relates to the common way addicts express their experience of addiction; that is, as a mental obsession and physical compulsion. The mental obsession includes a preoccupation with the next drink, even if this might be a few hours, days or weeks away. Even if an alcoholic athlete is able to abstain successfully during the lead up to an important contest, the obsession with the next drink is a constant. The physical compulsion refers to the phenomenon of 'craving' where the body takes the drink despite the intentions of the addict. The second (addiction – 2) varies more between addicts: it is the 'the addict's lifestyle' (Flanagan 2011: 282).

There is much more that could be said here by way of context and background, but it is expedient to move to the main thrust of this chapter, namely the life story of an addict. The story certainly gives us some more insight into what Flanagan means by addiction – 1 and addiction – 2, and how they manifest themselves in the life of a particular individual. There are countless biographies and autobiographies providing insights into the lives of addicted athletes, some of which I have mentioned already in this book. They contain the whole gamut of chaotic, humorous, tragic and shocking recollections of life as an addict and an athlete, usually a high-profile athlete. There are some who think that elite athletes are particularly prone to addiction.[1] There is certainly plenty of anecdotal evidence of addiction and/or other psychological problems among high-profile athletes, and perhaps the kind of personality required to achieve athletic success – that is, determination, obsessive training, ambition and so on – sometimes borders on dysfunction.[2] The following story does not have any of the glamour and glitz, but is a story of an ordinary aspiring athlete whose career and life were ruined by alcoholism. It also testifies to the complex range of personal and social issues that accompanied, or perhaps contributed to, the onset of addiction.

The story of George (a pseudonym) was relayed to me in a series of five unstructured interviews lasting over an hour each. George is an alcoholic in recovery who was entitled to treatment at the Sporting Chance Clinic in the UK, years after his professional football career came to an end.[3] He entered rehabilitation at a critical point and has been sober ever since, continuing to attend Alcoholics Anonymous (AA) and other '12-step fellowships' to help him stay sober. I have edited the transcripts to try to create a single narrative, but divided it up into sections to make it easier to digest. I have tried to keep editing to a minimum and present the story in George's words (including his frequent bad language and some of his most harrowing experiences), but I have sewn together five separate interviews, taken out questions and prompts by the interviewer, and cut down on the length in order to meet word limit restrictions for this book. I have removed any references that might threaten George's anonymity and have not corrected any factual inaccuracies or grammatical errors.

George's story

The early days and the identification of an 'ism': an underlying, or developing personality disorder

I am originally from Aberclwyd [pseudonym], a small rural coastal town in Wales with a population of about 2000–3000 people. I suppose looking back at the young me, I wouldn't have said I was necessarily shy *per se*, or at least I wasn't shy if I felt like I could be the centre of attention on my terms. I could be very shy around situations that I felt uncomfortable in, such as school. My talents were more creative; I was quite good at arts and crafts and design and technology. I wasn't academic, but I enjoyed and was good at most sports, and football became my main focus and was a good outlet for me. I felt different I suppose, whether that's true or not, I can't tell because I don't know how other people feel. I can remember the feeling of not being part of things, disjointed I think is the word. Although I felt part of being a team sometimes, I felt disjointed within that. Since leaving school, I have found out that I have a mild form of dyslexia. I couldn't read until I was 18 years old and never read a book before then. This caused problems in school because I would get panic attacks, worrying that the teacher was going to ask me to read in class. When this happened I used to just walk out of the class or throw something or get really frustrated. My mother protected me to some extent by writing letters to the school requesting that I wasn't to be asked to read out in class. This was probably counterproductive and didn't deal with the real issue; it was swept under the carpet in a way. This was just one example of my mother showing too much love whereas my father didn't show me any love. I feared him and built him up as this monster, but in recovery I've been able to understand him a little better – he was a very scared individual – and being a father myself I understand a little bit better about what was going on in his life.

When I was 11 years old I was sexually abused, by someone outside of the family where I used to work. I had several sort of small jobs when I was around that age and something happened on a few occasions which went on for probably a month or two. I told my mother about it and she said don't go back, but we didn't tell my father. Maybe I was a bit frightened my dad would have attacked him or something. There were other things that went on at that time which I won't go into because some of them are a little bit too personal, maybe a little bit too painful, but there were periods of uncertainty and real confusion when I was growing up. As I said, my dad was quite a physical person and he used to be quite controlling and domineering and I used to get ill-treated that way quite a bit. When I was about 11 or 12 the stresses of not wanting to be in school and then not wanting to come home because of the fear around issues in the house led me to my first addictive experience. I didn't feel I could talk to anyone about these things, and I don't know why I did it – I just used to go home and inhale gas from an aerosol in the toilet. I don't know to this day how I worked out how to do it because I never experimented with it with friends. Doing that was a form of escapism for me and I did it for a long time, probably a year or two. I don't know how I didn't end up with some kind of brain damage. My brother used to catch me occasionally and tell my father. But again, rather than asking 'what's going for you', or trying to understand, like I would do with my daughter, my father would tease me about it and sweep it under the carpet.

I also remember having this real fear of death and I didn't know where I was going to go afterwards and that used to scare the crap out of me, it really did. I had this deep feeling of nothingness, a real scared feeling and I was unable to vocalize this stuff – not being particularly intelligent, frustrated and trying to get these things out. I couldn't speak to my mother and father because I felt they would brush it off. I am not trying to justify their behaviour, but they didn't know any better. I've spoken to them about these things since so it's not an issue now but at the time it was very much 'don't talk about that' or sweep it under the carpet. Football was my outlet for all these things, but there were other things too, such as the aerosols.

When I was young I played a lot of football and it was important to me. We didn't have a great deal of money, but my parents always tried to get me the kit I needed and always took me to games or trials with a football club. I was a goalkeeper and as long as I had my goalkeeping gloves at the end of the bed, I was happy. In the summer holidays I would go down the football pitch with the other boys and I would play from 9 or 10 in the morning until 10 in the night and come back filthy. I used to hide the dirty clothes under the bed so my mother wouldn't see them. I would practice on my own in the garden if no one would play down the football pitch. Football was a massive influence in my life and I was determined I wanted to play professionally. There were 80-odd professional clubs in the league at that time in the late eighties/early nineties. I used to write handwritten letters to every single club asking for trials. I found one of the letters not too long ago and it was very simple the way it was written, 'can I have a trial at your football club please', it was like a child really. I think my mother would look over them after to make sure there were no spelling mistakes and stuff. I would re-write to those 80 clubs again and see if a scout would come down and watch me play.[4]

I can remember when alcohol first came into my life. I was about 8 or 9 years old and we used to go to my grandmother's house at Christmas and New Year, a woman I loved in my own little right – maybe because I felt she was somebody I felt at ease with. I used to just drink the cans of lager there and it lit me up in a way, it kind of made me feel quite, I don't know what it made me feel – made me feel okay I suppose. I can remember thinking afterwards; once it had gone I was gutted so when other people would go out of the room I was trying to drink theirs. Other than those occasions alcohol didn't play a part in my life until I was about 13. Then I used to go to beach parties, the typical teenage behaviour, asking people to go into off licences to buy us cheap alcohol. I was always trying to get off my face, and I just thought it was something that people did. If I'm honest I didn't like the taste of alcohol, I used to find it disgusting and had to work hard to drink it. Now and again my father would find me at beach parties, in a ditch with blood all over me and vomit everywhere. He'd throw me into the back of his van and take me home.

The beginning of a career in football

I signed with a professional club a huge distance from home at 16, right about the time my parents split up. I was very young leaving home and there were a lot of problems going on. Around that time my grandmother, who I was fond of, died and a friend committed suicide. The reality of life was kicking in, but I was still this dreamy person, as long as I could tip the ball over the cross bar in the last minute and save a penalty everything would be okay. By this time I had also developed an obsession with my weight because I was a little bit chubby as a child. I always used to get embarrassed in PE lessons when they used to ask us to take our tops off and I can remember feeling like I had these man breasts and a big stomach. It probably wasn't as bad as I thought, but in my mind I was this huge, fat, gross thing. I became obsessed with being fit and how I looked because I felt that if I had a good image about me physically then that would make up for all the other things that I felt that I lacked. When I started with the club, I was one of the most unfit to be honest, I was always at the back during runs, but in the second year of my apprenticeship I was at the front. Although I was a goalkeeper I realized it was important for me to be fit, but I became obsessed with it. I used to tell people what they should be eating. As long as I had my abs, my six pack [defined stomach muscles], I felt that I was better than other people I suppose. I used to think 'look at them, they're not fit, I'm fit, I've got this great body', blah de blah. I worked incredibly hard to maintain the physique, but in a very sick way. It wasn't just because I wanted to be fit, but more to do with my self-esteem and ego. I felt so crap about myself that I thought that if I created this ideal physical me, it would mask how I really felt. I can remember doing an obsessive amount of exercise. We used to live on the side of a mountain in this small terraced house and it had about 100 steps to the house and I used to run up them all the time. I bought a weights bench and me and my mate used to do weights and I was always doing press-ups. At the club the apprentices would arrive in the morning and prepare the kit for the professionals before our own training. In the afternoons we would do a shit load of running or weight training or agility work. We would go on gruelling runs – the thought of the amount of training we did makes me feel sick now. In the evening everyone else would be chilling out, but I'd go to the gym and train again and do more stuff. I would train three times a day, I was obsessed with it.

My drinking at the time had a certain pattern. I would train obsessively three times a day and then I would have a massive blow out on the piss. We would go out as a group of lads and go drinking but initially it wasn't that problematic. It was something all the other apprentices did. I was doing what most lads do, go on the piss, pubs and clubs, and stay out as long as we could, trying to find all the places that would stay open as late as possible. I can remember being in a particular pub and drinking a pint and looking at the bubbles at the bottom of the glass and getting that feeling, that glow, thinking 'this is alright this is, this feeling's good'. The taste of drink was fucking foul, I really didn't like it, but I worked hard to acquire a taste for it. As I got worse with my drinking, the drinks that I put into me were incredibly strong. It was about getting a hit. It wasn't about the taste for me, ever. I was going out looking for opportunities to be rebellious, mischievous, do different things and have a bit of fun, the usual stuff. The problem at that time was not how much or how often I drank, but more how I felt inside. I don't know how others feel, but I certainly felt all these strange feelings like, I'd exposed myself, I'd made a fool of myself and I was second guessing everything trying to work out what had happened. I'd internalize everything, trying to work out what others were thinking of me. I used to go into my head and feel very lonely, very isolated, all this shit and guilty crap and all these negative emotions, it's horrible, horrible feelings. At that particular point I think most people would have thought I was kind of odd. I was either a mad, centre-of-attention-type person, or quiet and intense and dark.

I don't remember any specific rules about drinking. Occasionally when we had games they would say you can't go out drinking, but I don't really remember it being something that was brought up that much, because we did it in our own time. I think it would be vastly different now there are expectations of footballers. I do remember getting constantly told off for my behaviour, but that wasn't neces- sarily always alcohol-based stuff but more to do with my arrogant sort of cocky way of being. If we turned up pissed up and performed appallingly we'd get pun- ished, but I can only remember one or two incidents like that. It certainly wasn't a regular occurrence. I would get into trouble for other stuff. I can remember the manager saying to me 'make me a cup of tea, the tea's in there, I want sugar as well', all this stuff, and I said to him 'well do you want me to fucking drink it for you as well?' He sent me out on the track and made me run round the track for hours. He didn't like me, and when he released me from the club I could see a wry smile on his face. I think he was, in some way, relieved to get rid of me because I was a complicated person. I was quite mischievous in some ways. I can remember getting kicked out of college – we had to go to college 1 day a week – for doing silly things. I won't give too many examples of those things, but just stuff like being cheeky and answering back. Very disrespectful in all honesty and it didn't go in my favour.

We had quite a good youth team at the club and we'd win most things to be honest, but even if we won 8–1 I'd be hard on myself for letting that one goal in. I can remember in one game I made a mistake and we lost 1–0 and that fucked me up for ages. I kept re-living it and re-running it in my head constantly. I just couldn't let it go, it would take me ages, I used to beat myself for ages about that. It was important for me to get it right I suppose, important for me to do a good job, maybe I wanted everyone to praise me I suppose and to say that I was good at what I did. There was a lot of dishonesty and deceit with me around not wanting to get told off. Although I hated the prospect of being told off, I acted in ways that led to it, not just with drink but with my behaviour and my attitude at times.

The end of a short career

Eventually I got released from that club after 2 years. I had an opportunity to go to America for 6 months to coach. I was disillusioned with playing football in the UK and thought going abroad would change things. A few of us went over, and boy did that open my eyes to life. It was before the 1994 World Cup and football was a big thing at the time. Back then, football was just developing, particularly in certain areas in America. When we arrived we were met from the airport by a limousine, which did my ego no good. There was a kind of press conference for players that came over and a big fuss was made of it all. The Americans might do this all the time, but for me it was 'fucking hell, this is amazing', and in my head this is what life was about. I didn't see it as a fantasy world, I thought this was how life is, or how my life is. And maybe a little part of me felt underneath that this is what it should be like, what I deserved, especially after the disappointment of being let go by the club back in the UK. The set-up was pretty unprofessional really, from the standard of the equipment we got to the expectations in terms of our time commitments. We stayed with families or in hotels, but everything was paid for.

Drinking was part of the life. We would drink when we could, not regularly because you were restricted sometimes because you stayed with families who frowned on alcohol. In fact, some of the states I went to were dry states, we had to smuggle booze in from other states to try and get some drink and when we partied, God did we party. I remember one particular nice family I stayed with whose kids we coached. One night I went out with some lads and got very drunk. I don't remember getting back to the house, I must have blacked out because I came to realizing that I'd wet the bed and was trying desperately to hide it by washing the bedding in the washing machine in the basement. I didn't know how the hell to use it but I was trying my best. The next thing I know, I'm upstairs with the husband's hand around my throat; he was kind of choking me. I must have blacked out again because I can vaguely remember doing things, but somehow I was in their bedroom and what I'd done apparently is actually pissed in the handbag of the wife. The husband really went nuts on me, I'd come out of this blackout state and he was shouting at me calling me a dirty bastard and all this stuff. I got reported, but didn't get kicked out of the country although that family didn't want to see or speak to me again. My drinking, I suppose, was slowly developing, but I was bingeing rather than continually drinking daily because I still had commitments. But it's not necessarily about my drinking and antics because maybe lots of young people do that kind of thing, it's more about how I was feeling inside about myself. It was embarrassing really. Before I came back I met a religious family; they were kind of born-again-Christian types. They would take me to church and they would stand up and sing hallelujah and all those types of things, and I used to get really embarrassed and I'd sit there and just think 'what am I fucking doing here'. But part of me realized that they were very kind people. They took me to Florida with them for a break and they were trying to encourage me to stay over there to take up a scholarship. At the time I had a girlfriend over in the UK who I didn't want to be with if I'm honest, but I knew I had to go back. I didn't want to go back, I wanted to go and live this fucking high life or whatever it was I was building up in my head.

When I came back from America I signed with a semi-professional club, but in all honesty my football-playing career started to fizzle out at that stage. I wasn't playing every week and I just had this one match, one game, it was in a cup that we played and we lost 3–0 and every goal was my fucking fault in my head. I had a nightmare of a game; I don't know why, I just did. And after that match I just thought I don't want to do this anymore, I'll do what I want to do type of thing. I thought there was more to life than football and if I'm not going to play at a good level then I'm not going to play at all. That's an example of my extreme thinking: fuck that I'm not playing if it's not going to be a decent level. Then I went on a mission to try and fill that void. I had this thing in my head that I was going to go to America again, visit this kind family on the pretence of taking up a scholarship, but what I really wanted was to get out there, go to LA to be a movie star. This is how my head started to unravel. My reality was far from the picture in my head. I was doing lots of different menial jobs, including working in a shop and as a doorman. By this time I had started martial arts, two different forms, kick boxing and karate. I got a black belt within two and a half years. I was around 20 at the time and in a relationship. She fell pregnant, but I wanted to go back to America. She threatened that if I did I would not be allowed to see our daughter and that I should get my priorities right. I did go to America, but it was a letdown, and I came back to my partner and we got married, bought a house and all that. I was very resentful about it all and stressed by the commitments that stopped my free-dom to live the life I wanted.

I couldn't cope with all this stuff that was going on, being married and all these different things. I was working as a doorman, doing the martial arts, I was doing well in that, super fit again, but then I would be drinking crazily. I also started working in leisure centres because my wife didn't want me to be a doorman, and started doing acting work because the other doormen were doing stints as extras on TV. In the leisure industry everyone seemed to be having affairs and on the piss all the time. I was doing around 80 hours a week and I loved the job in a way because it was all a laugh with the boys getting drunk and enjoying ourselves. I started getting very irresponsible, not going home or turning up drunk to look after my daughter. Looking back on it now, I didn't fit into that life, I still had that feeling inside of me that although I was with the boys and having a laugh I still felt part of nothing. I couldn't stand being in a relationship with the arguments and the fighting. My daughter was tiny and she was growing up and I was in no fit state to be a responsible father, I couldn't be what my ex-wife wanted me to be. I was providing financial support to a degree, and the drinking wasn't that bad initially, but there were periods where I was using alcohol, staying out and not coming home and turning up to work quite drunk. I used to go on all-day drinking sessions and sometimes not go home for weekends. Eventually it came to a head and I left. I was about 21 and we'd been married 6 months or so.

For a month I stayed with a guy who worked at the leisure centre and just went on fucking mad sessions. Although I went back to my ex-wife for a couple of months it wasn't working so I ended up leaving her again. During this period I started getting into trouble with the police. I was quite handy with my fists and I got arrested for a nasty assault on someone. The guy I was staying with kept a letter from the courts to say that the charges against me had been dropped. He kept it for weeks. I was only a kid and lived in fear, thinking 'fucking hell, I'm going down for this'. He eventually gave me the letter and said he just wanted to see me panic. I also assaulted a female colleague at work. I bit her as a joke, but as usual for me I took things too far. I ended up getting a final written warning on my record, having to go to a tribunal, having to stay away from that place for a month. Drinking was affecting my thinking and clarity of mind and making me a bit crazy and paranoid. Even so, I managed to build up a good CV because when I do jobs, I do tend to do them quite well because that's part of my nature. I can't stand being judged so I'd rather do things well. Unfortunately, when drink's involved, it makes it very difficult to keep this up.

The progression of the addiction

It was now clear that drink was becoming a big problem. A friend's mother was a counsellor and suggested I ought to watch my drinking. I still had this infatuation that I was going to be this amazing kind of movie star in Hollywood. I couldn't stand living the way my ex-wife expected me to live and I felt trapped. I was always sitting away in dark rooms listening to depressing songs and drinking beer getting into an almost morose, nice mindset that I could escape from the reality of my life. It was very confusing and still is to a degree. I then went through a phase of living rough where I was going from people's floors or sleeping in doorways or in people's cars and all these different things, I just lived this bizarre life really. I was homeless; I had no responsibility really other than turning up for work if I had to, and seeing my daughter occasionally, and it got quite messy with the courts around that time. And when I talk about this it makes me feel sick, because there is so much to say, so much to talk about, and the only way I could deal with it was to drink. So as long as I had my drink I could function to a degree. I ended up going back to America. I remember telling my daughter that I was leaving. She was only about three or three and a half. She was crying her eyes out saying 'where are you going Daddy?' and I couldn't understand why she was crying. All I felt was she was stopping me from doing what I wanted to do. And I remember saying to her 'what you fucking crying for? What's wrong with you?' That's how fucked up I was. That's how self-centred and selfish I was. I said to my ex-wife I'd pay my maintenance, and I did send money back for a while. It was horrendous in America; I was absolutely pissed up all the time. People were covering for me. I even missed the flight out there because I didn't look at my ticket properly because I was pissed up the night before and stuff. In my mind, I wasn't going out there to coach football I was going out there to jump over to LA and be a movie star.

I came back early and broke my contract because I missed my new partner. I had met her before going back to America. I also missed my daughter if I'm honest. I remember one of the kids out there giving me this teddy thing and I made out that I'd bought this teddy for my daughter, but I didn't have any money because I'd been pissing it up all the time I'd been there. I posted it through the letter box. If I look at it through a kid's eyes I just don't know what she would think of her father. We have a good relationship now, it's developed as a result of being in recovery, but fuck me, I was just a selfish fucker really. I stole a load of stuff while I was out in America, I thought, fuck you if you're not going to let me come home early I'll take all your stuff with me. Anyway, a family I was staying with paid for my flight home. They were a nice family and I said when I got back I would post them the money, but never did.

When I got back I worked in this place, in this hotel, this private club. I had nowhere to live, I had nothing because I had sold everything before I went out to America and didn't even get anywhere near LA to be a movie star. I was back living in people's cars, people's floors all that sort of stuff again. My friend who got me the job started to move away from me because I was getting a bit odd, my mental health was going. When I was 24 I ended up having pneumonia from my drinking. I was on a high-dependency ward in the hospital for 13 days and incredibly ill because of drinking and not looking after myself. As soon as I came out of the hospital I bought 20 fags and a bottle of vodka, it was the first thing I did, which was typical of me by that point. By this time, my drinking had gone from more sensible types of drinks like beer, well it was always strong beers, to spirits, because I wanted to drink as much as I could. At some points I was drinking probably 2 litres of vodka a day. I wasn't always drinking all day and to some extent I was still functioning and going to work. But the work that I was doing, on the door, meant that I worked at night and could snort coke or take some kind of drug such as amphetamine to keep me awake. I had a couple of shifts in a gym, I was a fitness instructor training people and I was off my fucking tree, it was ridiculous really. I was quite open about it and I told people I was an alcoholic, but there was no comeback because I think they were scared of me if I'm honest. I was a big guy and I was ugly looking, sometimes I'd have a shaved head and I looked scary, I suppose, to people, although I had a charm to me as well. I was very sort of aggressive and I had this aura of 'don't fucking come near me' but I could be quite cheeky. I was a master of trying to manipulate every situation for my own good. I didn't do anything at work, I just stood there, and as I got worse and worse I ended up just not doing my job really. I would turn up on shifts, see if there was enough staff, and then go and watch a football match or do something else. My partner didn't know where I was half the time.

Although I knew that alcohol was a problem for me then, I just carried on the life I was leading. I can honestly say though that I've always known there was something deeper than alcohol. The way my thinking had always been and the way I felt was very odd. I couldn't stand feeling a certain way, riddled with fear and constantly on the move, running from things, and alcohol was the thing that worked to keep things at bay and stop my racing brain. It still races like fuck today, you know, but I look after it differently now. I was always looking for answers to this bigger question if you like, of life, and drinking fuelled that for a long time. It also helped me to contain things if you like, but then it stopped working. I'd portray this almost cardboard gangster image, this hard man. I was around all these guys who probably felt just the same as I fucking did but just play the game like everyone else. Maybe they don't feel that way, but I couldn't deal with my feelings of that stuff although they would never know that because I wouldn't allow them to know that. I didn't understand it back then, I thought this is how I was supposed to be, this is who I am, you know. But I didn't have a fucking clue who I was. I used to brag about my exploits sometimes because that was the bullshit bravado that, 'listen to this story', 'I slept with a girl last night' or 'I beat this guy up and he deserved it' and all this sort of shit. I didn't always end up beating people up. I can't say I enjoyed violence and the next day I would think about it, but I thought it was all part of being a tough man.

By the time I was about 24 I had been drinking daily for probably 3 years in all honesty and maybe a little bit longer really. I'd gone from a type of person who could drink whenever I fancied drinking, to drinking vodka and spirits. I also took drugs, was on anti-depressants and was going regularly to a community alcohol team. Sometimes when I was out I was doing bizarre things like staring at the wall for 2 hours in the club after taking ecstasy. I was kind of mad really, and people would ask me 'are you ok?' and I'd go 'fuck off, leave me alone'. Eventually, I had to stop working on the door because it got to the stage where I was drunker than the people coming in the club itself. I was high on cocaine and different drugs to control the effects of the booze because I was trying to keep my job. My partner at the time, who I'm now married to, bore the brunt of a lot of this insanity; the chaos, the changing jobs and the constant moving. I think I've moved about 26 or 27 times in my life. My wife and her family did take me in for a little while and I just sort of slept in my wife's parent's house, but then we got this flat together for a couple of years. By this time, I had kind of given up work in a way. I was doing some acting work and different stuff occasionally, but she used to go to university and hold down two jobs while I would just stay at home and drink. The daily drinking of vodka meant I couldn't work or do anything the same anymore, and things were getting worse and worse, the blackouts were horrendous. Before this point, I could quite easily drink maybe 2 litres of vodka, but at about the 25–26-year-old mark I couldn't drink as much because I was blacking out quicker.

My behaviour was chaotic. There were these two lads who lived in the flat below us and they were kind of noisy. I used to throw rubbish bags from outside at their flat and bang their door, and I could hear them saying, 'God this guy's fucking nuts', you know, 'don't open the door to him'. They were just young lads playing music, smoking different stuff and I did find myself a couple of nights going down there and smoking opium with them. I was erratic and used to do stuff like that when it suited me. If they were noisy when I didn't want them to be I'd go fucking nuts. After they left the flat, two other lads moved in and they were pretty similar, they were drinking a lot and noisy and that. For some reason our key would open their flat door and one night they had come in and I could hear them and I could smell burning. I'd drunk a half bottle of vodka and said to my wife 'I got to get some more'. I went to the off-licence and come back and I could smell the smoke even worse. It was about 10 at night and I went downstairs and let myself into their flat downstairs. There was smoke coming from the kitchen so I walked through, and flew into this psychotic rage. I threw this thing which was burning on the stove through the window, smashing it. Another time my wife came back from work one day and I would be hanging out of the flat window by my feet virtually, ready to drop myself on my head. She is only small and would try to pull me back into the house. She didn't know, when she came back, whether I was going to be on the floor, drunk or dead, basically. Although I never beat her up physically, the psychological abuse I used to put her through was unreal you know. My brother rented a flat about three or four streets down and he suspected that something wasn't right. He said to me recently that sometimes he'd pop round and he'd see bottles of vodka, and he'd think, 'fuck I'm going to get away from this fucking lush, this loony'. One night I manipulated him into buying me drink because I didn't have any money. Sometimes I'd get drink from a local shop on tick [on credit] but he bought me some. I had this breakdown, this real meltdown where I just completely started crying, and then I went outside and I literally jumped on a car. I was a big heavy guy then and I was jumping on the roof of this car like the hulk, it was bizarre and then I'd fall off and roll on to other people's cars going into the middle of the road, and cars were swerving past me and I would be on the floor crying and be trying to punch people as they walked past. My brother didn't know what to do so he phoned my wife who was working, she had to come and get me and the two of them then took me over to the hospital. On the way I opened the car door and started head butting the floor as we were going round a roundabout, literally trying to scrape my face on the floor. When we got there I was rolling around on the floor crying and again trying to punch people when they walked past. They put me in this wheelchair and they sent me to this room in the hospital. I sat in the sink, like a loon, just sat blubbering in the sink and I was throwing equipment at the nurses. They wouldn't come near me. The following day they booked me to see the psychiatrist in the local mental hospital. I had another breakdown a little bit later on and by the time I was about 26–27-ish, I was seeing psychiatrists, going to half way houses because I had tried to take an overdose twice.

I was given diazepam as a home detox. I think I must have had about 30–40 tablets, and I took them all with a bottle of vodka and ended up not being able to move from the sofa for about 4 days. I'd started going a bit yellow as well, and blood tests showed my liver was starting to get affected. I ended up having to go to places to get tablets given to me with the street drunks. I was going down to this place to pick up medication, I had to have a breathalyser test before I went in this halfway house, and I had to have counselling there as well, and it was bizarre because I found out later there were AA meetings in this building and I'd never been introduced to AA at all, you know? No one suggested I go to AA meetings, but I did have acupuncture there. I used to just sit with the street drunks and play pool with them and get my tablets and off I went.

I was going to this community alcohol team as well so I was trying all this stuff to stop drinking. I did manage to stop for 6 months and got into drama school. Unfortunately I started drinking again. I thought, if I just have a couple of bottles of beer, I'll be alright, type of thing, the usual shit that I hear these days. Within a week I was on a bottle of vodka again. Somehow I got through the year-long course at drama school. I think drinking helped because I don't think I could have done it sober because the fear in me was unreal. I would do the drama school bit, drink a bottle of vodka in the evening, get up, go to drama school, drink the bottle of vodka, and it was just a cycle of that for ages, and I used to say to the tutors that 'I can't help that I'm drinking again', in drama school it's like, 'well fuck it, who doesn't drink'? Drinking was part of the culture, but I don't think they realized quite how bad I was, particularly the insanity of what was going on. Anyway, I got through the course and I passed it, but then when I stopped at drama school it was weird because I thought well, now I've got an agent I don't have to do anything, so I just sat at home and drank.

The last year and a half of my drinking I went to a place where I can't really describe. I was living back at my wife's parent's house because we could no longer afford the rent on the flat. Any money I earned went on booze. I would use the banks, I would use my wife, I would use the shop, I would use my mother, I would use anything I could to drink; I'd steal, I'd sell drugs, I'd do things like that. My wife used to go off to her job and do her stuff and I used to drink. By this time I was drinking in the morning, so I'd get up and I had this little routine. My father-in-law used to have cans of lager at the side of this cabinet and underneath this cabinet there was Jack Daniel's and rum. They would go off to work, I'd drink two cans, that would give me the courage to go out and buy vodka and I had to buy another two cans to replace the cans I'd taken. If I couldn't drink the lager, I might lie on the floor and sip out of his rum bottle listening to see if anyone's coming and then fill it up with a bit of water so no one would notice. Sometimes I would black out and drink the Jack Daniel's bottle and my wife would have to replace it with a brand new one the following day.

The blackouts by this time were horrendous. Once I came out of blackout hanging off the edge of a bridge. I was trying to kill myself. It's a bizarre thing, because until I went to AA I didn't really understand blackout. I thought it was a natural thing to do, that all people who drink got them. I used to be around people and I'd say to them 'I can't remember some of the night' and they would say the same, but these blackouts would last sometimes days and weeks where I just couldn't remember anything and yet I was functioning. One time I got in in my wife's mother's car in the morning, drove up to the gym where people saw me on a treadmill, looking and smelling like a tramp. I drove back home and to this day I don't remember any of it. My wife says that in the end I'd have a drink and after the first two or three mouthfuls I would verbally abuse her, yet I don't remember a thing. I was still doing things in blackout, but my brain had switched off. To this day, there are lots of things that people tell me happened which I can't remember. It's very embarrassing and makes me cringe. When I woke up I had that terrible 'I've done something wrong' feeling; constantly towards the end it was 'what the fuck have I done now?'

Although I never physically assaulted my wife I couldn't really predict my behaviour when drunk or in blackout. If I had continued drinking who knows what would have happened. I used to tell my wife that I would kill her parents, and accuse her of sleeping with her brother. My head was so sick I'd look at the weather man on TV and think he's better looking than me so she must fucking fancy him. I would give her a fucking hard time all night saying that I'd chuck the fucking TV out the window; you are having an affair with that fucking weather man. I was so fucked out of my head, and the poor woman believed a lot of this shit, towards the end she was like a fucking wreck because I was so convincing. I can remember grabbing her arm once, and I can remember I went to kick her. I don't know if I would have been violent towards her if it had continued. In therapy I had to look closely at my behaviour towards my wife. A therapist said that when you're drunk and you have sex with a woman and they're scared of you, it's a form of intimidation. She wouldn't really be free to consent because of the power I had over her. I was horrified when he said that because we did have sex and I never felt I was forcing myself upon my wife, but if she was scared of me then she was probably doing it to avoid my anger. All I can say is that if you are an alcoholic like me and have the same sort of tendencies, same thoughts and same sickness in the brain, then it's impossible to rule anything out. My conscience didn't work when drunk. I was very violent towards people, and who knows what might have happened. I am very lucky because my wife saved my life in a way. She has told me that she used to wish that I would die because I was in so much pain. She didn't mean it in a callous way, it was just she didn't want me to be in that pain anymore. In the end I was physically very ill. I was pissing blood quite regularly now, shitting blood, coughing it up, I mean I was so swollen, and by this point, just before I went to treatment, I was 19 stone 10, my face was yellowy orange, I looked like a pumpkin head, my head was like a fucking basketball! Fucking so fat and my head was massive, I mean, my toenails were black, fucking disgusting, gammy you know, I didn't wash, I stank of arse, you know, I was just like a tramp, I don't know how my wife still fucking fancied me! She probably didn't. My wife put up with so much shit.

Rock bottom and recovery

I was still pursuing ways to get help, counselling and stuff, and I was almost addicted to them. I wasn't the type to hide it, in a way I was like, 'I've got this problem, fucking fix me', you know. I remember going to this counselling thing and next door to it was an AA meeting. The counsellor knew I was an alcoholic but he didn't suggest going to AA. That was the second missed opportunity to go to AA. Eventually, I had this meeting with a friend of my wife's in work who knew somebody who had been to Tony Adam's Sporting Chance clinic. I'd kind of exhausted all avenues where I lived and I knew that I was running out of options. I tried all these alternative therapies like reflexology, acupuncture, Reiki and all sorts of shit; not shit, they're good stuff, but they didn't work when you are drinking the excessive amounts that I was drinking. Anyway, I was broken and when I say this time I was physically fucked, I was physically fucked. Something else inside had gone this time, you talk about your soul, mine was fucked – it was like that candle that flickers and it's almost going out. I was on the brink, I didn't want to die, but I didn't want to live. The jumping-off place, rock bottom, and without doubt I couldn't continue. I would have killed my wife, killed her family or killed myself. Physically, I don't think I had much left in me either, I was starting to pack up and I was only 30 years old. It's sad really, to see such a person who still thought at this point he was a professional footballer. I was deluded. Reluctantly, I contacted the clinic, but was worried that I had to stop drinking even though it was killing me. I had to go away for 28 days, and start getting real I suppose, and start growing up. My wife insisted that I phoned the clinic and after a couple of days of procrastination I did. I had to go to London and get assessed by a psychotherapist and he said in that meeting, yes, you are definitely one of us. He was an alcoholic with many years of recovery that had obviously experienced a lot of this stuff as well. They said I should go in as soon as possible. One of the conditions was that I had to make sure that I didn't drink for 3 days prior to going, which strangely wasn't as hard as I thought it was going to be, although after the 3 days I was in a real mess. I was shaking uncontrollably, hallucinating and sweating horrendously. But it seemed that a little chink of hope had come in and I really put the effort in to stop. I had stopped taking drugs about 5 years previously. I didn't carry on because I guess I wasn't a drug addict. I wouldn't take coke unless I was drinking. I think alcohol was my drug of choice if you like, not that you choose to go to the places that went with it, but for me, alcohol was the Rolls Royce. I also smoked cigarettes and different things like that because I do have this obsessive mind, but for me alcohol was the primary drug. I'm prone to secondary addictions, but in recovery, in order to be sober of mind, I have had to stay away from those other things because if I put those things in my body I will end up back where I started: it's been proven time and time again.

I had my first real experience of AA in treatment, and we had to go every night and had to start working through the 12-step programme. The guys that ran Sporting Chance, well the main therapist and the guy who ran it, were both in recovery themselves. I can remember how cynical and sceptical I was of therapy, group therapy, psychotherapy, alternative/complementary therapies and everything. We had to see a trainer, eat, clean and all these types of things, and it was incredibly intense. The facilities were quite extravagant. When I was having therapy, halfway through the sessions I just used to say, 'okay, I've had enough now', and kind of walk out, and the guy, the therapist, used to say, 'I fucking tell you when you've had enough'. I admire him now for challenging me but no one had ever done that before. I used to say to him 'talk to me like that again I'll take you outside and fuck you up and we'll be scrapping'. One of the guys in there used to say I was one of the angriest guys that he had met in that place. I don't know whether he says that to everyone but the therapist used to call me the rebel without a clue. I was just this person that was quite rebellious but I kind of wanted to get well but I didn't want to do what was required. We had to do things like wash our own clothes and I hadn't done that for years. I had to learn how to do things again. Even going to the toilet was strange because most of my craps for the last years were blood and liquid because of all the vodka I was drinking. When I stopped it, I kind of got constipated for days upon days, it was horrible. I can remember having my first shit after about 8 days. Anyway, me and this other guy used to go to these meeting and I used to take the piss and we used to laugh ourselves to sleep at night. After 12 days he left because he had this thing in his head he was going to go home for his daughter, but I knew he wasn't, he was going home because he had had enough and he wanted to drink. So it was me on my own in the middle of nowhere in this like, little cottage-type place, having therapy 6–8 hours a day and having to go to AA meetings every night.

I remember I was so scared, we'd have carers in one cottage and I'd be on my own in this other one. I used to check every single fucking cupboard and door was locked and everything because I thought some fucker would be hiding in the cupboard and was going kill me at night or something. I was petrified sleeping on my own there. It was only towards the last week or so I was allowed to contact people. My wife came to see me and I could see the relief and happiness on her face because she could see I looked so much better. She had to sit with the therapist and have a session herself, and we had to have therapy between the two of us – that wasn't too easy to be honest. I came out after 28 days; they gave me some information about AA meetings around the area I'm from. I can remember feeling 'oh my God, what the fuck, I'm back out here in the real world', and I was scared, really scared. We had a barbeque to celebrate me coming home, and I said to my wife 'I can't do this, I feel like shit'. The frustration, anger and real resentment that I had to do life again was very strong. Looking back, I guess I just wanted to go to rehab, stop drinking for a little while, and then carry on. I realized I couldn't drink anymore – something happened in me, something had shifted in me – there was no way I could go back because I would be dead pretty soon. And I didn't want to die either.

After leaving treatment, I went to my first AA meeting at this place that I still go to quite regularly now. I was supposed to have done these three steps of the AA programme in treatment, and to get out and get to meetings and stuff. I was still attending the community alcohol team for counselling and different things, I had couples counselling with my wife, and I was having aftercare in treatment. I was just going to about one AA meeting a week. I had to overcome the panic and all this confusion that I had. I tried all sorts, I tried working like mad to do different jobs, to do anything, but avoided the 12-step programme. After about 10 months I can remember just lying in the corner of the room screaming at my head to shut up because I just couldn't handle this racing brain which alcohol used to stop. When I stopped drinking it just became faster and faster and I didn't know what to do to stop it. I used to panic and scream at my head, I used to say things like 'shut the fuck up' because I couldn't handle it, and I used to smash the house up when my wife was in work. I hated it. I didn't want to drink again because I knew that that was going to kill me but I felt like I was going to hang myself. I remember headbutting the door and the wall about 20 times, and my head was pissing with blood, because I just wanted my head to shut up, it was fucking horrible. So I started increasing the meetings and I started talking to people in recovery and asked for help. I had a guy who helped me massively in my second year of recovery; he introduced me to AA properly and helped me understand what the fellowship of AA was about. In the 12 or 13 months or so since leaving rehab, I hadn't progressed beyond the first three steps. I realized afterwards you don't just do them, you have to continue to work at and live them in your life. So this person spent probably a good 2 years with me, about 3–4 days a week, for 3–4 hours a day, and we used to go to meetings and spend loads and loads of time together. I used to get all this crap out that was holding me back and stopping me from moving on in life, I suppose. I was quite untrusting still, although I liked this guy I didn't want to share my step 4 and 5 with him.[5] I was about 2 years in by now, and it took me about 7 months to write it [step 4 and 5], and I decided I was going to go back to treatment and share it there. This therapist was later my best man at my wedding and I'm still in contact with him now, he's a good friend of mine. My pain wasn't immediately taken away; in fact, it was a while later when I got to step 7 that this stuff started to release in me. It was like a release, like I had forgiven myself in a way, it was a strange feeling of peace. I went on to work through the first nine steps, making amends and different things, and that released a lot in me. The tenth, eleventh and twelfth steps, are about living now really, and I try and apply them in my life, so that's a big factor of why I don't drink today. Treatment sort of stopped me but AA keeps me sober if you like, and I need to do that probably for the rest of my life. I used to go to two meetings a day but now it's probably about two or three a week, I help people now myself, you know, I do service in AA. I help people by doing step work with them and lots of other things. I can contribute and give back what I was given – my life back – although the life I had wasn't really a life, I suppose. I don't want to go into what AA is about too much, but it helps me massively. Once I found this AA thing, you know I'd tried everything else, I realized that I couldn't fuck around with it, this was going to be a way out. Instinctively, not in my head because my head used to tell me a pile of shit, but instinctively I knew that this was going to save my life and up until, you know 8 years on, it has. I've fought and I've kicked and I've screamed and I've not wanted to do any of it but I've stayed sober and that is the main thing, that's what AA tells me, providing I don't pick up a drink and I live in the day the best I can, I have a chance. It doesn't mean my life's going to be wonderful, it just means that I don't have to drink. I used to think AA would fix everything in my life, but that's not the case.

My mother and father never saw much of my drinking but they could see a massive change in me. I can see it these days now in the way that people look at me, the relationships that I have, the respect that I feel off them – it's not fear anymore and dread, I could see it in their face, it's different, there is a love there now that's healthy and not fear-based. Sometimes the unspoken things are far more powerful than actually what's been said. I think my daughter was too young to understand fully what was going on because she was 9 at the time, but as time went by I could see and sense in her that she could see that this person was changing in front of her. It was scary for her because I was this depressed, dark person, and all of a sudden I had a bit of hope and I could see she liked it, but it unsettled her as well.

I've looked at all the other addictions if you like, as well. I stopped smoking, stopped caffeine; I stopped behaving badly with food and all different things. I was very heavy at one point in recovery and I ended up losing about 6 or 7 stone and got back to a kind of fitter me. I started excessively training and doing things like running a marathon a week. I don't know, I was almost existing on this, they call it a 'self-will' in AA where it's just a drive to just do things, and nobody sits still, and even when I wasn't doing it my head was racing. I was working as an actor and when I wasn't acting I was doing support work and I got myself on this counselling course at university. The day after my first day on the course I found out I had bowel cancer. I don't know whether I brought this on through stress, whether it triggered it, whether it was the food I was obsessively eating, all the abuse I'd put my body through with all the drink or if it is a genetic thing. I had to stop university, I had to stop everything and that's what happening now. I've being trying to get well from the cancer and it's been fucking hard to be honest, but I haven't thought of drinking or anything. I sometimes want to fucking escape. I can't, I can't run away from these things. I have to face it, and it's been a real tough time through treatment, and a lot of setbacks, everything really. I still do what I need to do for AA, with my AA stuff because of my head, but also, like I said, I thought that might maybe help me with everything else. I have had to have additional therapy to help deal with cancer and other issues. To have bowel cancer at 36 is quite young, but I remember my daughter saying to me, 'why you', and I said, 'well, why not?' Everyone else has shit in their life and she was angry I suppose, in her own way.

I think, to be honest, everything that I have done in my life, even at the age of 11 and 12 when I was inhaling gas on my own and stuff, is part of being an addict. I don't think anyone really knows that but that's how it seems to me. I don't know how other people felt but how I felt was I didn't feel part of anything, and all these things I think are contributory factors to my alcoholism. I'm not trying to segregate and say that these feelings are unique to an alcoholic because some of the stuff I talk about is part of the human condition. Human beings have these things, these feelings I think, it's just the extreme sensitivity that I've always had in me. A lack of acceptance of the world and life and holding on to things for far too long, way past their sell by date. I think once I put a substance in me, that addictive substance, this obsession of my mind and an allergy in my body starts off that cycle in motion. I don't think people who are not an addict or alcoholic or whatever have that because they can have a drink and put it down. I can't deal with life very well, and a lot of people can't who are not alcoholics as well, but the point is, is that if I deal with it in the way that comes natural to me, I die. Simple, and that's not dramatic, that fucking happens all the time so I have to look at ways of dealing with life in a different way and AA does that for me. The other things haven't really come close to that to be honest.

Looking back

I was brought up not to show weakness and all that type of thing, 'tough men don't eat quiche', that sort of crap. I wouldn't have had the humility back then to ask for help even if it was available. There is more awareness around this stuff these days and I think culture has changed; I think there are facilities and different things that people can access. I think that even the whole type of attitude, if you like, around therapy, is a lot more open-minded now than it was back then. I think I was afraid of saying 'I need fucking help for my head', in case people thought I was nuts. I had no idea, no concept about mental illness or addiction. I was just doing my life, I didn't have any awareness about these things, I was a fucking child. I've had help, massive help throughout my life, and that's been through people, it's been through institutions, it's been through all this different stuff and I don't mean just mental. I'm on about any type of facility that is available to helping people like myself. Maybe I could have gone to somebody at the football club; I couldn't have gone to the main manager but certainly some of the coaches. I warmed to certain coaches and would have been able to maybe say 'look, is it okay to feel this way?' It all depends on the person, there are certainly some I wouldn't have given them the time of day even if they offered to help. They didn't realize I had a problem. Like I said, the drinking was apparent, but that's what people would do, blah di blah. It wasn't easy for them to recognize that I had deeper issues. I didn't have a head that was a greenhouse that they could look into me, and because I didn't tell them anything, I just would be arrogant or I would be sort of cocky or bolshie or whatever word you'd want to use – quiet, moody – I would not allow others to get near me in that respect. It wasn't the same as it is now – they have therapists, they have life coaches and they have all these different things because people are aware of the pressures that come with playing at that level.

If I put myself in the shoes of young football players now and imagine how I would react if someone like me went to talk to them as part of an education programme or something, I would be doing something to crack jokes or just wouldn't take it seriously. I'd have thought that's you, not me, I would have had an arrogance about me so I would expect that a lot of people would have that attitude in that setting at that age. I would imagine, I don't know. But I remember in another situation later on in my life people used to do that regularly, people from an industry would come in and used to talk about their experiences and stuff as I'm going through this thing, and I used to think, 'fuck off you fucking dick', you know, and I would have thought – 'that's your life, what do you know about mine?', sort of thing. Real narrow mindedness, I wouldn't have heeded any warnings. So if I'm like that – not saying every human being is that way – but if I'm like that I imagine there are some who would be similar. Maybe there would be some with a bit more humility than I had and engage with the process. I didn't engage in anything, I couldn't sit still. I would imagine that most people would want to just play football – not hear about some alcoholic footballer's life. Maybe if they were in a bad situation where they'd stop playing football and they had to find some sort of help because they'd got into addiction or alcoholism or whatever, maybe they would listen then. But even in recovery there's been many times when I don't listen, I think I know better. It normally takes a lot of pain and suffering before I change, I don't have foresight; I only have hindsight, and so generally have to go through these experiences. Then I kind of reflect and learn from that. I don't see what's coming my way really, suppose if I did I wouldn't get out of my chair, I'd be fucking too scared.

When I look back at my career, I think it gave me a focus until it ended, but I think that drinking and using would have always been there. Although I drank when I was playing, the fitness side of things and the obsession of trying to be the best and all those types of things, kind of kept it at bay more – I had more of a direction, more structure and all those types of things, but when that went from my life the inevitable was going to happen. I think if I didn't have that football, sometimes, I don't know whether I believe this, but sometimes I think it – you know, I played professionally for a football club and ended up in a clinic that was linked to football – a treatment centre which started my recovery. It makes me think if there is a direction in life that is mapped out – not that I know this – that maybe my purpose solely for playing football was to get well through the treatment. Maybe it saved my life in that respect.

Summary

This is one story and each story is different, but as Flanagan (2011) suggests above, there is a common phenomenological experience to addiction. There is a drive to use, and we have seen that this is associated with a range of problematic emotions or difficulties which will vary from individual to individual. This desire to use becomes so powerful that the alcoholic uses alcohol in ways that lead to a variety of problems. Some are related to a loss of control from being drunk, others are related to the chaotic lifestyle around active addiction and others are the physical consequences of excessive drinking. Active addiction is ugly and there are inevitable victims. There is nothing glamorous or heroic about it, a fact that only very few are prepared to point out lest they be seen to be disrespecting or tarnishing the sacred image of some of our most talented, but deeply flawed athletic heroes. The journalist Johann Hari, writing in the *New Statesman* soon after George Best's death, asked: 'Why do we honour a violent thug?' Hari offers a counterpoint to the 'fawning obituarists' who he says ignored the significant flaws in Best's character in their rose-tinted tributes.[6]

Redemption and recovery is possible and addicts can change through a variety of means. Pickard and Pearce (2013: 166–167) argue that:

> . . . addicts use substances to cope with the psychological distress associated with personality disorder and other psychiatric conditions, and will continue to do so unless they learn alternative coping strategies to manage negative emotions, address underlying issues, and gain opportunities for a better life, containing positive, alternative goods.

For George, recovery eventually came by being introduced to 12-step programme of AA while in rehab.[7] Rehab is not a quick fix and there are many different approaches. What they seem to have in common is that the addict must engage and participate in their recovery. They must want to get sober, but it is not an easy journey.

Notes

1 http://www.castlecraig.co.uk/blog/05/2015/sports-and-alcohol-addiction-unlikely-link (accessed 8/05/2015).
2 See Gogarty and Williamson (2009) for an interesting overview of athletes and 'their demons'.
3 The Sporting Chance Clinic (http://www.sportingchanceclinic.com/) is a rehabilitation facility started by the former footballer, Tony Adams. It provides treatment services for current and ex-professional footballers for a range of different addictions and other issues.
4 The route to professional football in the UK at the time, and which still exists to a certain extent, was that talent scouts (employees of the football clubs) would go and watch young boys play football for local clubs. If they were impressed with what they saw, they might invite the boys to come for a trial at the club. If the boy did well at the trial it might lead to an opportunity to go to the club as an apprentice. This in turn might lead to a professional contract, but the reality was (is) that there is a very high attrition rate. Only the select few get a professional contract, and only a few of those go on to a career in football.
5 He is referring to the fourth and fifth steps of the 12-step programme of AA. Step 4: Made a searching and fearless moral inventory of ourselves, and step 5: Admitted to God, to ourselves and to another human being the exact nature of our wrongs. http://www.alcoholics-anonymous.org.uk/About-AA/The-12-Steps-of-AA (accessed 8/05/2015).
6 http://www.newstatesman.com/node/152132 (accessed 21/05/2015).
7 For a discussion about how AA works, see Flanagan (2013).

References

Flanagan, O., 2011. What is it like to be an addict? In: J. Poland and G. Graham, eds. *Addiction and responsibility*. Cambridge, MA: MIT Press, 269–292.

Flanagan, O., 2013 Phenomenal authority: the epistemic authority of alcoholics anonymous. In: N. Levy, ed. *Addiction and self-control*. Oxford: Oxford University Press, 67–93.

Gogarty, P. and Williamson, I., 2009. *Winning at all costs: sporting gods and their demons*. London: JR Books.

Nagel, T., 1979. *Mortal questions*. Cambridge: Cambridge University Press.

Pickard, H. and Pearce, S., 2013 Addiction in context: philosophical lessons from a personality disorder clinic. In: N. Levy, ed. *Addiction and self-control*. Oxford: Oxford University Press, 163–189.

Conclusion

My aim in this book was to make a contribution to the debate about the problematic relationship between alcohol and sport. I have argued that alcohol is a toxic psychoactive substance that brings about a number of harms, both to the individual and to society more broadly. Despite this, alcohol use, and on occasions its abuse, remains prevalent in many cultures. Youngsters are initiated into drinking alcohol by their peers and adults, including teachers, coaches and parents. No other psychoactive and toxic substance is treated in this way. Alcohol use and misuse are normalized.

Sport plays a key role in normalizing alcohol consumption in a number of ways. It provides a platform for alcohol companies to market their brands and even provides a troubling loophole in marketing regulations aimed at protecting youngsters from being exposed. Many alcohol brands are linked inextricably with sport. Many countries have outlawed sport sponsorship by alcohol companies and there is a growing demand that a total ban on alcohol sponsorship of sport be introduced. Watching sport and drinking alcohol go hand in hand and alcohol companies seek to capitalize on and further strengthen this link. There is a price to pay for this relationship in terms of health and social problems associated with fans drinking too much alcohol. Sport also highlights the link between celebration, alcohol and excessive drinking. It plays a key role in reinforcing the practice of getting drunk as *the* method of celebrating.

Despite sport's association with health and fitness, many athletes including elite athletes engage in heavy drinking. There is an alcohol ethos that promotes heavy drinking, particularly at certain times. Although governing bodies and coaches may set rules about drinking, it is clear that the experienced ethos is at odds with these ideals. Evidence shows that athletes often get drunk sometimes with, or sometimes without, the blessing of coaches. Athletes are no different to others in their age group in that when given the chance they choose to party and to drink. Athletes – particularly, but not exclusively, elite athletes – are in the public eye and are 'role models'. They should not exemplify irresponsible and reckless alcohol consumption and the problems that go along with it. Their behaviour further normalizes alcohol and contributes to the creation and maintenance of a problematic alcohol ethos in sport.

There is an argument that problems associated with alcohol are caused by a few individuals who lack self-control. The alcohol companies in particular subscribe to this idea. It is true, relative to the numbers who drink alcohol, that only a minority have problems, but this is a significant minority. Far more people are abusing alcohol than admit to it. Moreover, even small quantities of alcohol alter the minds of drinkers and put them at risk of 'acting out of character'. Once drunk, we have diminished control over our actions so getting drunk should be discouraged. The prudent thing to do is not to reduce one's rational capacity through alcohol. This does mean educating individuals, but it also requires a change in the drinking culture or ethos. Such a change is by no means easy. Researchers and health professionals have been trying to combat the alcohol culture for years. It is a slow process, but it involves a complex set of measures including education, reduction in availability, closer regulation of alcohol supply, good role models and a change in the way alcohol and being drunk are perceived. I have no easy answer to the question about how the ethos can be changed, but change it must. Numerous reports, research projects and policy documents, some quoted in this book, suggest a number of strategies for reducing alcohol consumption. The overwhelming message is that alcohol is too easily available, is too cheap and is promoted too heavily and that drinking is deeply ingrained in our cultural practices. The problem is not just about a few 'bad apples'.

It is the case that some individuals may have more serious problems with alcohol. It is true that certain athletes are recidivists when it comes to alcohol-related offending. I have argued that the first offence should be considered a 'red flag', an indicator of potential dependence or addiction. The US model of punishment and some form of therapeutic intervention is good practice. If the athlete is rehabilitated and does not offend again then the intervention has worked or the incident was a one-off. Either way the outcome is good. If they do reoffend, it might be indicative of more serious issues that require further therapeutic intervention. There is no guarantee that therapy will work. Individuals have to buy into the process, but punishment alone is ineffective in changing potentially disordered behaviour. Disordered drinking is often 'normal' drinking in sporting cultures, which makes it more difficult to recognize and to help individuals who may need it. This is further grounds for reforming the ethos.

There have been many examples of athletes who have had serious alcohol problems during and after their careers. Some have become long-term chronic addicts, others have recovered. Addiction is a complex condition that has emotional, psychological, genetic, neurological and social aspects. There is no single cause, but drinking alcohol is of course a necessary condition. The more alcohol is consumed in the general population, the more alcoholics there are. Sport should take alcoholism seriously. We discourage drug use, in part because of the threat of addiction. The threat of alcoholism does not carry the same fear yet a minority of drinkers will go on to become alcoholics. There are a number of other risk factors that predispose certain individuals more than others. The more we know about alcoholism, the more we can help prevent it and help those who suffer from it. Again, this requires a significant change in attitude towards alcohol, heavy drinking and addiction. It is a condition that causes suffering not only to the addict but also to their family and others. Addicts can recover in a number of ways, but invariably it requires the help of a community where alcohol use is not routine, normal or encouraged. I hope this book at least gets those involved in sport to think more carefully about alcohol and its association with sport.

Index

AA *see* Alcoholics Anonymous
absenteeism 11
abstinence 42, 88, 103
accidents 10, 12, 17, 63; *see also* fatalities
Adams, J. 35
Adams, Tony 63, 88, 106, 113, 142, 149n3
addiction 4–5, 9, 19, 109, 113–120,
    151–152; brain processes 110–112;
    choice 113–114; compulsive behaviour
    107, 112, 113; compulsory therapy
    124–125; diagnosis 120–124; George's
    story 130, 131–149; personality
    disorders 108; phenomenology of
    128–130, 148; punishment or therapy
    118–120; responsibility 114–118, 119;
    stages of 123; young people 50; *see also*
    alcoholism
advertising 3, 28, 31–35; bans on 17, 18,
    31; outside schools 44n11; *see also*
    marketing; sponsorship
Agassi, Andre 61
age of drinking, legal 21, 32
agency 65, 78, 111
aggression 3, 27, 33, 38, 81, 123; *see also*
    violence
Albers, A.B. 22–23
Alcohol Concern 35, 44n11
alcohol industry 16–17, 151; influence on
    policy 14, 18–19, 36; marketing 27–36;
    regulation 33; resistance to change 6
Alcohol Use Disorders Test (AUDIT)
    120–121
Alcoholics Anonymous (AA) 7, 109, 121,
    130, 140, 141, 142–146, 149
alcoholism 4–5, 88, 108–126, 151–152;
    brain processes 110–112; choice

113–114; compulsory therapy 124–125;
diagnosis 120–124; George's story 130,
131–149; phenomenology of addiction
128–130, 148; punishment or therapy
118–120; responsibility 114–118, 119;
see also addiction
alcopops 22–23
Anderson, E. 55
Anderson, P. 32
Andrew, Rob 95
anger management 119
Anheuser-Busch In Bev 28, 29, 30, 36
anti-social behaviour 10, 11, 33, 39, 55,
    123
anxiety 7
Aristotle 75–76, 79, 85–86, 97–98, 112,
    114, 115–116
Armstrong, Lance 81–82
Arnett, J.J. 50
Arsenal FC 40, 49, 55, 84
Asquith, Herbert 7
athletes 47, 63, 150; alcoholism 118–125,
    130, 151; celebrating with alcohol
    39–43; college sport 53–55; elite sport
    55–62, 67; offences 93–94; personality
    disorder 107, 108; punishment of 4, 91,
    95–96, 102–103; role models 4, 73–75,
    81–89; youth and community sport
    52–53
AUDIT *see* Alcohol Use Disorders Test
Austin, E.W. 32
Australia: alcohol industry 19; cost of
    alcohol 12; fatalities 9; rugby players
    59; sponsorship 29, 30; violence 11;
    youth and community sport 52
autonomy 98, 99, 101, 124